H$_2$O

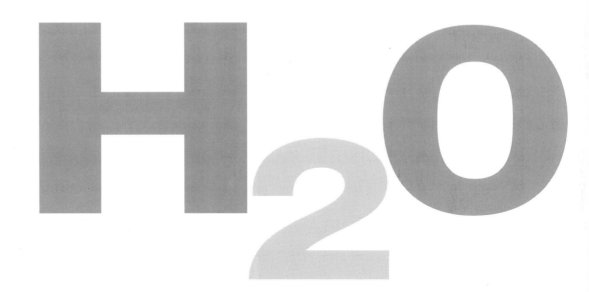

Healing water for mind and body

Anna Selby

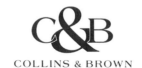

COLLINS & BROWN

First published in Great Britain in 2000
by Collins & Brown Limited
London House
Great Eastern Wharf
Parkgate Road
London SW11 4NQ

Distributed in the United States and Canada by Sterling Publishing Co.
387 Park Avenue South, New York, NY 10016 USA

1 3 5 7 9 8 6 4 2

British Library Cataloguing-in-Publication Data:
A catalogue record for this book
is available from the British Library.

ISBN 1 85585 7448

Designed by XAB
Editor: Mandy Greenfield

Reproduction by Media Print UK
Printed and bound in Poligrafico Dehoniano

SAFETY NOTE
The information in this book is not intended as a substitute for medical advice. Any person suffering from conditions requiring medical attention, or who has symptoms that concern them, should consult a qualified medical practitioner.

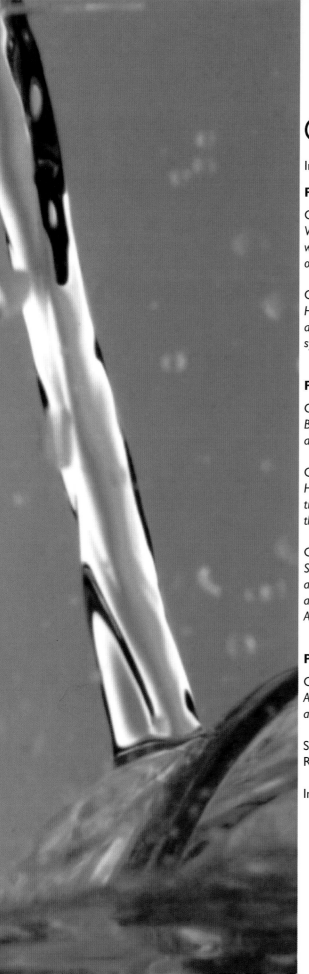

CONTENTS

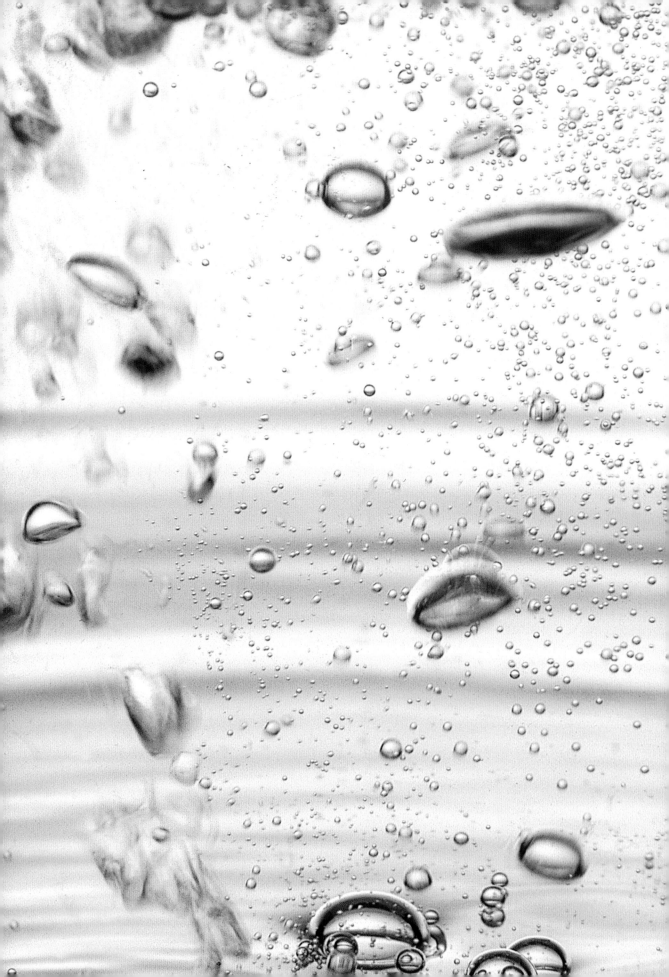

INTRODUCTION
PURIFYING WATER

Water is synonymous with purity, and its cleansing properties are far from being merely physical. Every one of the world's great religions uses water symbolically for the purification of the soul. Think of the pivotal Christian rite of baptism or the holiness of water to Islam. And at the dawn of prehistory, our ancestors often made their shrines at the point where a spring bubbled up from the ground or within a cave. It seems that water matters to us almost as much as a means of spiritual purification as it does as a way of cleansing the body, both within and without.

Even for those who do not adhere to a particular religion, water still casts a unique spell. Perhaps it is the magical qualities of water – that most adaptable of substances, able to transmute from liquid to solid to vapour – that have always fascinated us. Perhaps it is the fact that our bodies comprise around 75 per cent water – so like is attracted to like.

We are drawn to water and refreshed by it. Being by water calms and energizes us; being in water relaxes and strengthens us. This book explores the benefits of using – both within and without, for mind and body – the last great underexploited resource that lies all around us. Water.

CLEANSING WATER

Water cleanses – a simple and obvious fact. But from this one idea, humanity has conjectured for millennia on the properties of water, which is both refreshing and purifying, renewing to body and soul. In baptism, water symbolizes rebirth. As part of a fast, water cleanses not just physically but spiritually. And water has been central to most of the oldest forms of health care.

The healing properties of water were recognized by the Greek physician Hippocrates (c.460–377 BC) centuries before the birth of Christ, but they were almost certainly known about and used long before then. King Solomon (c.1015–977 BC) and the Queen of Sheba built palaces on the shores of the Dead Sea to benefit from its therapeutic powers, while Cleopatra (69–30 BC) used its water and mud as part of her beauty regime. The Romans, of course, built baths over thermal springs just about everywhere they went. In the eighteenth century, spas – from Baden-Baden to Bath – became all the rage and everyone who could afford it went to 'take the waters'. In the nineteenth century, bathing in the sea became the latest fashion, with elaborate bathing huts on wheels to convey modest Victorian ladies into the water.

While people were taking these various water cures, they would have discovered that there were other benefits, besides those to their physical health. Energy levels increased, minds became simultaneously calmer and more alert, people were less vulnerable to stress. And while it would be logical to regard all this as a mere side-effect of having hydrotherapy treatment or a holiday by the sea, it has now been shown that such benefits are the inevitable result of rehydration. Simply by drinking more water you begin to feel better on every level. It may be rather harder to prove, but there is a wealth of anecdotal evidence that being by water is, for many people, in itself a spiritual experience. Think of the mesmeric rhythm of the sea, the utter tranquillity of a lake in the mountains, the exhilaration of a crashing waterfall.

If you cannot get to any of these natural wonders, you can always create your own by means of visualization. One of the simplest and most effective of meditation techniques, visualization is like a holiday for the spirit. You can buy audio tapes that use the sounds of the sea or conjure up pictures of it – these are widely available. Once you have the knack of meditating to a tape, you can then make your own and describe a scene, or use a sound, that you find particularly relaxing or beneficial.

VISUALIZATION TIPS

When you meditate in any way, your temperature drops, so wear warmer clothes (and ones that are loose and comfortable) than you would if you were just sitting. You need to be free from distractions, so unplug the phone and, if there are other people about, ask them to be as quiet as possible and not come into the room. If, however, there is someone else with whom to do the visualization, this can often prove beneficial, adding to the focused atmosphere. Sit on the floor with your legs crossed or sit in a chair – the most important consideration is that you are comfortable.

Before you begin, take a few minutes to settle yourself, both physically and mentally. Take three long, slow, deep breaths, concentrating on the exhalation so that your body feels quite empty before you breathe in again. You will have plenty of thoughts whizzing around, but simply watch them; do not get caught up with them. Place them on one side to deal with when you have finished the visualization. The actual visualization technique is explained in greater detail on pp. 132–3.

When the session is over, do not jump up immediately. Instead, remain seated for a few minutes, breathing slowly and deeply, and try to keep that sense of tranquillity for the rest of the day.

WATER, RELAXATION & MEDITATION

We are all drawn to water – perhaps because it is the element from which we, like all living creatures, emerged before the dawn of man's prehistory.

Even those people who do not like to swim or to be immersed in water usually enjoy the sight and sound of it. Waves tumbling on to shingle or the rhythmic splashing of a fountain have an instantly soothing effect.

The most dedicated urban dwellers find that the natural sound of water is, above all, calming. No doubt this is one of the reasons why overwhelming numbers of people go to the sea for their holidays. Water makes us relaxed, playful, happy. In a world that releases ever-increasing stresses upon us all, these are qualities we need not only to appreciate, but to harness.

CALMING WATERS

Whenever on holiday and by the sea, make the most of the calming power of water. If you can, swim every day. Try to get to the water when there are fewer people around – especially early morning and evening – and simply walk along the shore, letting the water lap over your feet and ankles. Paddling is not only pleasant and relaxing, it stimulates the circulation. If you have trouble sleeping, walking at the water's edge is particularly beneficial, promoting a deeper, more restful sleep.

Listening to the rhythms of water reminds us at the deepest level of that time of ultimate warmth and security in the womb. If you are staying near enough to the sea to hear it from your bedroom, keep your window open wide. You will certainly benefit from improved sleep. When I spent a year living in Polynesia with my young son, among many other wonderful discoveries we found the best place to sleep ever. We lived in a house with no walls on a beach in Western Samoa, where you heard two levels of water music simultaneously. There was the crash of ocean on reef and the susurration of the waves of the lagoon on to the sand. We never had a problem sleeping.

WATER MUSIC

The sea, streams, waterfalls, steady rain – all have this power to soothe away stresses and still the mind. You can, though, enjoy these benefits without leaving home if you find room for a fountain. This does not have to be on the scale of a Moorish palace or the Trevi fountain. You can buy a small fountain – for indoor or outdoor use – at most garden centres, which costs very little, is easily assembled and can run off the mains. The sound of a fountain has the effect of instantly lightening the atmosphere. There is a wide variety of sound styles to choose from – pebble fountains, cascading fountains or simple china bowls. I've seen them work beautifully not only in the garden, but in hallways, reception rooms and bathrooms.

STILLING THE MIND

The sound of moving water on its own can be a potent force for stilling the overactive mind. Just sitting by the sea, a stream or a cascading fountain will often bring a sense of tranquillity but you can also increase the effect by using relaxation techniques or by meditating on the sound of water. (This is explained in more detail on pp. 132–3.) If you can be by 'live' moving water

while you meditate, then so much the better. If not, there are numerous relaxation and meditation tapes available using the sounds of the sea and those of sea creatures, such as whales, that are also remarkably calming and effective.

WATER WISDOM

Like the ocean, your body's fluids are a salty cocktail, spiked with precious minerals, such as gold and magnesium.

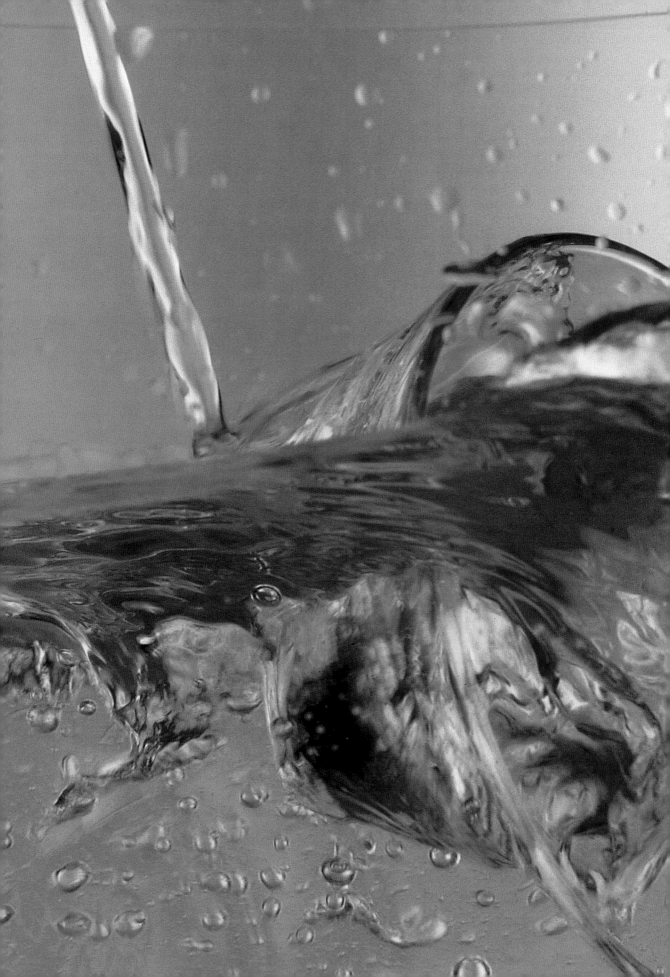

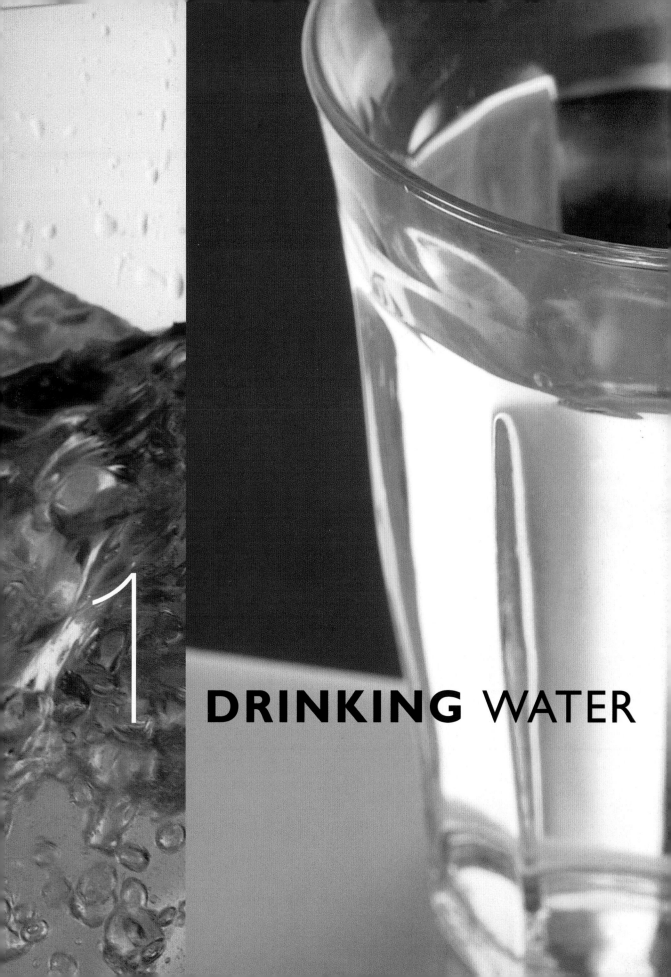

1 DRINKING WATER

THE LIQUID OF LIFE

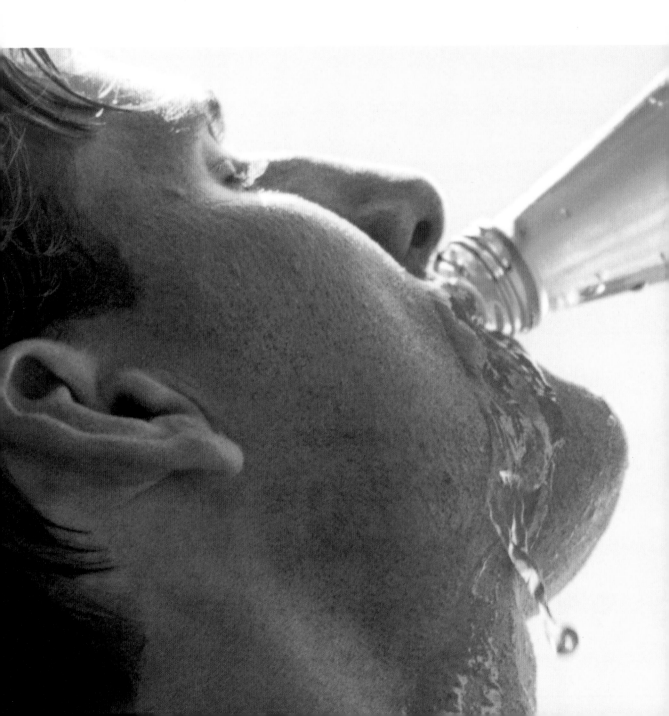

Water is essential to life. We can go for weeks without food, but without water we die in just a few days. And while few of us are likely to face death through lack of water, the vast majority of us are sufficiently dehydrated to cause damage to our health.

According to a study carried out in 1999 – the *Volvic Hydration Report,* undertaken on employees in 100 workplaces – dehydration affects both the mind and the body. We begin to feel thirsty at 1 per cent dehydration, and by 2 per cent our ability to work starts to diminish. At 4 per cent dehydration we start to feel lethargic, apathetic and bad-tempered, and we become more vulnerable to stress; feelings of nausea set in. Death occurs at 20 per cent dehydration. But, *even before we notice feelings of thirst,* water loss can affect the normal functioning of the body, making us more susceptible to stress and reducing the ability of the immune system to fight off disease.

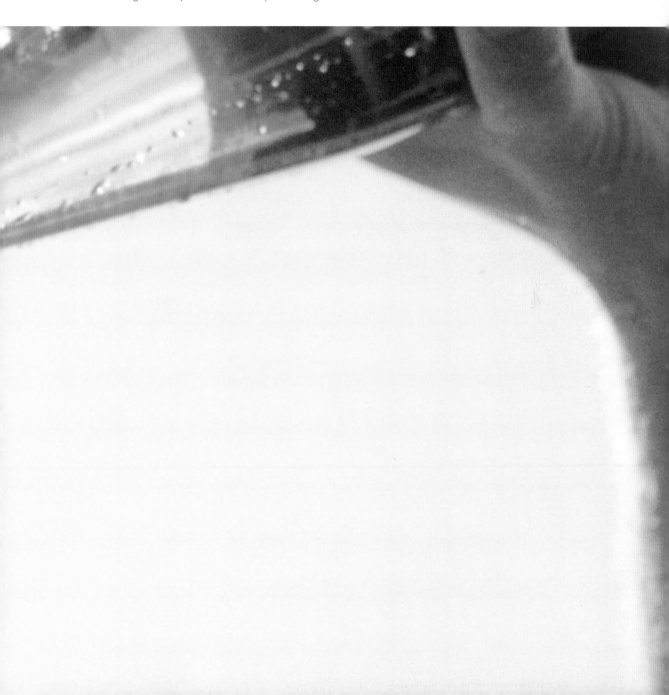

THE WATER CURE

People have been using water for their health for centuries, and from the very earliest times the connection between water and health must have been clear. There are a number of signs that indicate we are not drinking enough water. Skin is one very visible indicator and it can be affected in a number of ways. It may become flaky and dry and it is more likely to get lined and wrinkled.

If you are prone to skin conditions, such as eczema or psoriasis, dehydration may make them worse. Another very visible sign is urine, which becomes darker and thicker if you do not drink enough. If you are drinking enough water, it should be almost colourless. Headaches can be caused by dehydration – though, of course, they can result from other problems too. Mentally, dehydration can make you unable to concentrate or think clearly and you may feel tired and rather disengaged from life, too.

The earliest forms of health care would have evolved over the course of years, based on observation and empirical treatments. And water played a pivotal role in all such early medicine. In different times and different places in the world – from Egypt to China, and from Rome to India – water has been seen as vital to health and the water 'cure' has taken on numerous forms. Water treatments have been used both to treat specific ailments, particularly digestive and muscular disorders, and as a prophylaxis – a general preventative against illness. Water has been used internally and externally, and frequently a cure would involve both types of treatment.

Different types of water have also been used. From the earliest times, the water from hot and cold springs and the salt water of the sea were both used to improve health. The high salt and mineral content of the Dead Sea meant that nothing could live in it (thus giving it its name), but gave it its celebrated therapeutic powers and made it a focus of the ancient world. Cleopatra, for instance, made use of both its water and its mud in her beauty routine.

The Greek physician Hippocrates, too, prescribed spring water for internal and external treatment 400 years before the birth of Christ, as well as using healing treatments – not dissimilar to those used in hydrotherapy today – to emulate fever as a method of overcoming infection.

WATER WISDOM

Many of the indicators of dehydration – dry skin, dark urine, lack of concentration – occur before we even feel thirsty.

ROMAN BATHS

It was the Romans, however, who institutionalized the idea of water as a health cure. Throughout the Roman Empire communal baths were built and became central to the life of the town, a sign that however far-flung an outpost it may be, it was truly civilized. Most Romans would visit the baths at least once a day, and one begins to grasp their importance to the Empire when one learns that in the fourth century AD, in the city of Rome alone, there were almost 1,000 public baths. Mixed bathing was regarded as scandalous, but nevertheless became increasingly common until a rota was introduced in the first century AD. Men usually went in the late afternoon or evening, while women used the baths in the mornings.

The early baths generally had three principal rooms: the *apodyterium,* or dressing room; the *tepidarium* or warm room; and the *caldarium,* or hot room. Usually there were also *laconica* (very hot rooms), *frigidaria* (cold plunge-baths) and exercise facilities. These might include covered walkways, running tracks, swimming pools and gymnasiums, exercise courtyards or covered halls in chillier climates (such as Britain), where people could weight-train or undergo massage and beauty treatments. In the more elaborate baths there were places to sit and chat, shops, even libraries on-site, making them in effect the complete leisure centre of the ancient world.

Exercise was usually taken naked, with the body covered in oil. After exercising, the Romans would go first into the *laconica* and sit there until they began to sweat – in effect, with its intense dry heat, the precursor of the modern sauna. Next, in the more humid *caldarium*, they would clean their bodies by scraping off the oil and dirt with a *strigil*, a small metal or ivory tool. After this they would spend a little more time sitting in the *tepidarium* before

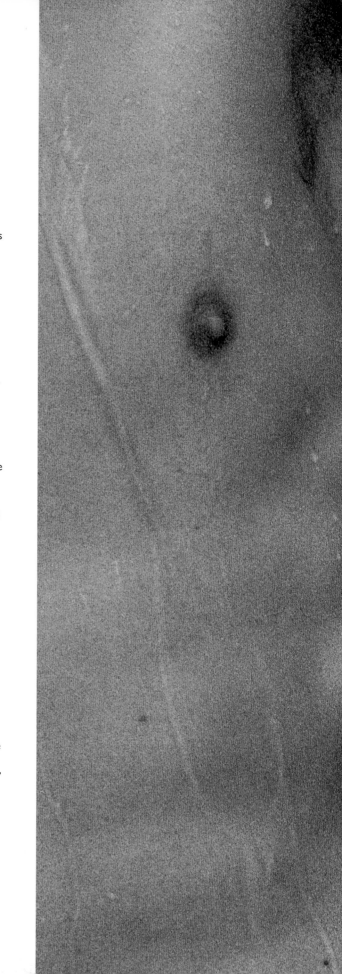

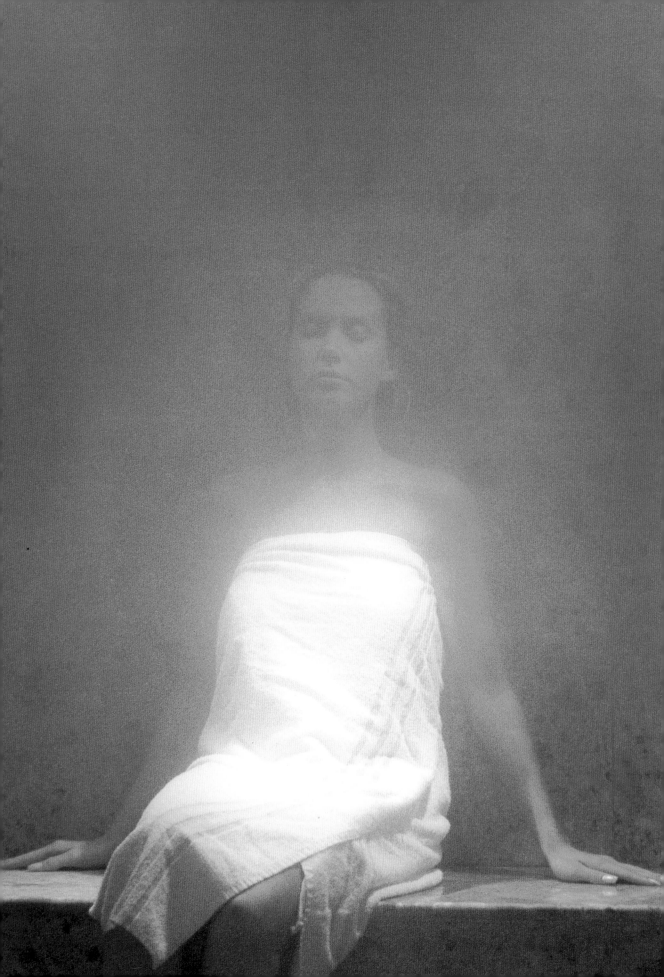

plunging into the *frigidarium*. The hot rooms were heated by a charcoal brazier at first, but later an elaborate system was introduced in which a furnace would heat up air, which then passed through vents in the walls and under the floors.

SACRED SPRINGS

Even by the standards of Roman baths, some were exceptional, as in the case of Bath, in England, built because of its hot springs and sacred long before the coming of the Romans. The fact that water came gushing out of the earth at 118°F/48°C and at a rate of more than 200,000 gallons/1 million litres a day must have seemed a natural wonder of phenomenal proportions to the early Britons. However, the Romans, too, were sufficiently awed to build a temple there to Sul Minerva, goddess of healing and wisdom. The Romans certainly recognized the healing powers of Bath's waters, too. They built a vast and luxurious complex around the original spring, including a steaming swimming pool and a cold plunge-pool. An inscription from the Greek lyric poet Pindar (c.522–440 BC) over the Pump Room reads, 'Water is best.'

While some of the original Roman building remains, much has disappeared under the rebuilding of Bath in its second heyday. The eighteenth century saw a huge revival of interest in the healing powers of water and, all over Europe, people travelled to spas, where they would take an annual cure. Sometimes this was because they suffered from specific ailments, but often it was simply the thing that educated people did – and it became as much a social event as a curative one.

THE FIRST HYDROTHERAPISTS

As the popularity of spas grew, so the number of treatments on offer inevitably expanded. In the eighteenth and nineteenth centuries, hundreds of European towns became famous for the healing powers of their waters or the particular methods of their leading practitioners. Many of the hydrotherapy treatments available today were invented during this period.

In the first half of the nineteenth century, Vincent Priessnitz (1799–1852) was one of the pioneers of hydrotherapy, based in Silesia. His rather spartan cures using only cold-water treatments became famous throughout Europe. Pastor Sebastian Kneipp (1821–97) devised somewhat kinder treatments using hot and cold water, which were so successful that there are still many centres today based on his work. By the end of the nineteenth century, hydrotherapy was becoming equally popular in the United States, particularly after Dr J. H. Kellogg (1852–1943) published his vast treatise, *Rational Hydrotherapy*, which explained the various treatments available and how they worked.

Throughout much of the twentieth century the healing powers of water were somewhat forgotten, while the world marvelled at the very different approach to health care epitomized by the modern-day miracles of insulin and antibiotics. However, all over the world, traditional spas have continued to work quietly and effectively behind the scenes. In fact, in many countries (particularly within continental Europe) water treatments are regarded as so successful and intrinsic to health care that they are available free under national health systems. Recently, however, people have once more been becoming increasingly interested in water and its protective, strengthening and soothing powers. It looks as if the water cure is on the verge of its next rebirth.

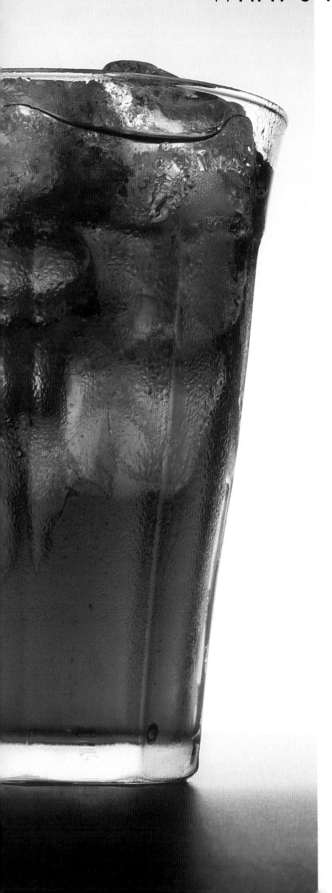

WHAT'S THE ALTERNATIVE?

Faced with the facts of general dehydration, the obvious solution is to drink more – but will *any* drink rehydrate? Unfortunately not. In fact, some of the most popular drinks will not only *not* rehydrate you, but will actually dehydrate you instead! The list of drinks that you should limit yourself to taking in moderation, or should cut out altogether, includes alcohol, tea, coffee and many carbonated drinks (except for fizzy water itself). This may sound rather daunting, especially if your favourite drink is on the 'forbidden' list. However, nothing is ruled out completely – it is merely a case of wise and occasional drinking. Rather than having several cups of coffee in the morning, limit yourself to one, and preferably not every day.

ALCOHOL

Alcohol dehydrates the body. Anyone who has ever suffered a hangover knows that one of its side-effects is a raging thirst. Indeed, there is a school of thought which claims that drinking 1pt/600ml of water after too much imbibing will prevent a hangover altogether. While that is rather wishful thinking, it will certainly dilute the unpleasant effects, because you have given the body extra water to compensate for the dehydration brought about by the alcohol in the first place.

Besides dehydration, there are other good reasons why alcohol should be taken only occasionally and in moderation. For the weight-conscious, it has the alarming properties of being very high in calories without offering any nutritional benefit. More importantly, it is well known that alcoholics tend to suffer from liver damage. However, even in people who drink just a bit too much a bit too often, the liver can be affected. There are toxic chemicals in cheaper bottles of wine known as aldehydes, which are also produced naturally within the liver as it detoxifies a wide variety of substances, including wine itself. It is these aldehydes that are responsible for those hangover headaches.

But the problem extends beyond headaches. Because alcohol brings about a double dose of aldehydes, the liver cannot process its detoxifying functions so successfully and there is an ever-growing build-up not only of aldehydes but also of other toxic substances, which the liver cannot deal with because it is so stressed. The end results of poor liver function are food allergies and intolerances (see below), fatigue, lowered immunity to disease and wide-ranging chronic illness.

COLA DRINKS

Most cola drinks contain caffeine (see Coffee, below), sugar and other undesirable additives. There are some carbonated drinks that comprise just water with added fruit or herbal extracts, but always read the label first so that you know exactly what you are drinking.

COFFEE

One of the more problematic characteristics of coffee is that it acts as a very effective diuretic on the body. This means that urination increases and not only do you lose fluids but at the same time the coffee robs you of such precious minerals as magnesium, which pass out of the body in the urine.

The caffeine in coffee has the effect of blocking vitamin absorption by the body. It also encourages the build-up within the system of one of the least desirable heavy metals, cadmium. Caffeine is, of course, best known as a stimulant – people rely on their morning cup of coffee to kick-start them for the day. However, it is also linked to raised blood pressure, with all its accompanying dangers, and it now seems that caffeine may also interfere with the way in which the cells of our body repair themselves on the deepest level – thus, in the long term, injuring our immune systems.

TEA

Tea contains tannin, the astringent also used in the tanning process of turning hides into leather. Tannin does not have a particularly beneficial effect on the body, either. Like coffee – which also contains some tannin – tea contains caffeine, which as we have seen is diuretic and has a dehydrating effect.

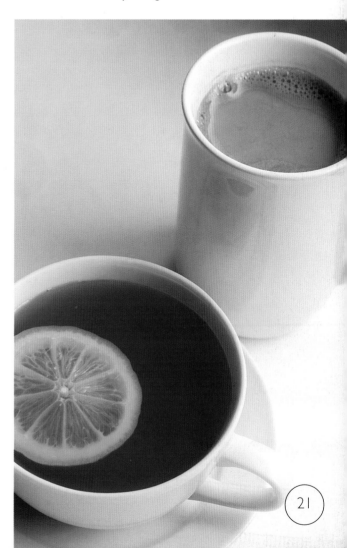

FOOD INTOLERANCE

One of the other problems associated with coffee is that it is so addictive. Once your body becomes used to the effects of caffeine, it needs more of it (just as with any other addiction) to give you the same boost and, inevitably, you increase the amount you drink. To complicate matters, such addictions are often simply the other side of the coin of a food intolerance.

A food intolerance is not the same thing as a food allergy. Allergies tend to result in a violent and immediate response to a particular food or drink, and in the worst cases can cause anaphylactic shock, when the throat constricts and the lungs fill with fluid so that breathing becomes difficult. In the case of a food intolerance, however, the reactions are not sudden but consist of one or more of a diverse range of long-term conditions, such as eczema, rheumatoid arthritis, digestive disorders, migraine or PMS.

The irony is that it is the very foods that are the staples of our diet that turn out to be the ones that cause the problems. In fact, those foods we crave – and coffee is a good example – are often the source of all manner of long-standing ailments. With hidden or masked food intolerances, the body not only adapts to the offending substance, but becomes dependent on it. The food is, none the less, acting on the system as a toxin and your body, unable to absorb it in the normal way, reacts against it. Problems may flare up elsewhere that seem quite unconnected to the problem food, especially as the reaction can take place several days later. Because satisfying the craving actually makes you feel temporarily better – that kick-start cup of coffee in the morning, for instance – identifying the cause of the intolerance can be difficult.

The only way to establish whether you do have an intolerance to coffee is to see what happens when you try to do without it. If you have been drinking increasing amounts of it, it is likely that you will have formed an addiction to it. This will mean, in the short term, that you might experience some unpleasant withdrawal symptoms. These most commonly may be a headache or nausea, but if you keep away from coffee for a few days, you should start to feel much better. If you are not addicted to it, you can, of course, have an occasional cup of coffee but nobody should drink it every day.

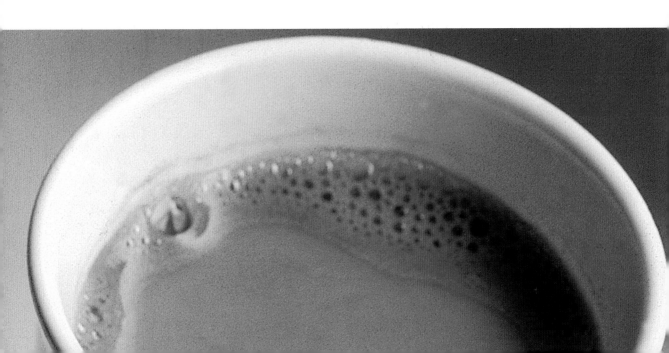

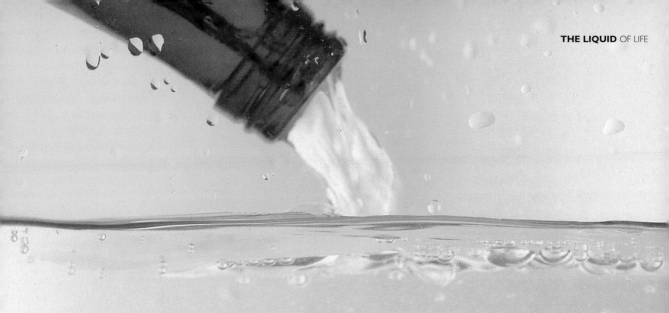

HOW MUCH WATER DO WE NEED?

Given that problems due to dehydration can occur before you even notice you are thirsty, what is the solution? The simplest and most obvious one is to drink more water and to drink it *before* you feel thirsty. On average we need 3$\frac{1}{2}$ pints/2 litres of water every day for optimum results, so you need to have this as a target and check throughout the day that you have had your quota. At first, you will probably feel that this is much more than you can manage and that you now spend the whole time rushing to the lavatory. However, you will be surprised at how quickly your body will adjust – and you will even start feeling thirsty if you drink any less.

SEASONAL CHANGES

You can lose 17–30fl oz/500–900ml of sweat every day and, when the weather is at its hottest, your water needs become greater, so it is important to replenish supplies all the time. In a very hot climate, it is a good idea to drink a large glass of water every hour.

DRY ENVIRONMENTS

If you spend a lot of time in very dry environments, you need to compensate for the resulting dehydration. Typical problem areas are overheated or air-conditioned offices and homes and aeroplanes. Drink at least one large glass of water every hour to compensate.

EXERCISE

Because you are likely to be perspiring more heavily during exercise, you will need to top up your reserves. Drink some water before you begin, during the exercise session itself (especially if you feel too hot, thirsty or dizzy) and when you have finished exercising. Depending on how energetic the exercise is, drink $\frac{3}{4}$–1$\frac{3}{4}$ pints/$\frac{1}{2}$–1 litre of water.

THE BEST WATER

Water is indisputably the best thing we can drink. But does that go for all types of water? Can we rely on what comes out of the tap to be a major benefit to our health? Unless we are particularly fortunate and happen to live next to a spring that is piped directly to our kitchen sink, the answer is that our tap water may be far from good for us.

Around 800 chemicals have been found to be present in drinking water. They may have originated in pesticides or weedkillers, in factory waste, air-carried pollutants or traffic fumes. Wherever they come from, they gradually find their way down into the water table and, from there, into our domestic water supply. Between 1985 and 1987 there were almost 300 known cases in England and Wales alone of pesticide levels in drinking water going over the permitted limits.

WATER CHART		MG PER LITRE
THOR SPRING ICELAND	CALCIUM MAGNESIUM SODIUM POTASSIUM IRON	4.5 0.92 11.5 0.5 0.03
HIGHLAND SPRING SCOTLAND	CALCIUM MAGNESIUM SODIUM POTASSIUM IRON	35 8.5 6 0.6 LESS THAN 0.01
VICHY FRANCE	CALCIUM MAGNESIUM SODIUM POTASSIUM	103 10 1172 66
BADOIT FRANCE	CALCIUM SODIUM MAGNESIUM POTASSIUM	190 150 85 10
SNOWY MOUNTAINS USA	CALCIUM SODIUM MAGNESIUM POTASSIUM	78 7 33 3
EVIAN FRANCE	CALCIUM SODIUM MAGNESIUM POTASSIUM	79 6.3 2.4 1.1

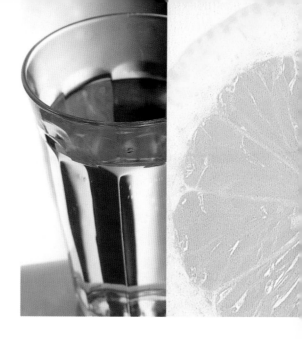

HYDRATION
DURING THE DAY

HYDRATION DURING THE DAY

7 a.m.	During the night, your body will have lost water, so drink a large glass (8fl oz/250ml) of water as soon as you wake up. This will also help as a detoxification aid for your kidneys and liver. Have breakfast at least half an hour afterwards.
9 a.m.	If your means of transport to work is dry, hot, overcrowded or stressful, then you will already have started to dehydrate. Take a bottle of water with you while you travel, or drink your second glass of water now.
11 a.m.	Drink a third glass of water now; more if you find yourself in a hot or arid environment.
12.30 p.m.	Drink a glass of water half an hour before you have lunch.
2 p.m.	Drink your fifth glass of water now to ensure clear thinking – this is a time when many people find that their concentration and energy levels dip.
4 p.m.	Drink your sixth glass of water instead of having an afternoon cup of tea or coffee.
6–7 p.m.	Have another glass of water as you leave work or when you get home. Leave half an hour before you eat.
9 p.m.	Drink your last glass before you go to bed, as you lose water during sleep. But do not drink it so close to bedtime that you have to wake up during the night to go to the lavatory.

UNDESIRABLES IN WATER

Unfortunately, all sorts of undesirables find their way into our drinking water and often we do not know about them until it is too late.

O Bacteria: although epidemics of cholera and typhoid are out of the question in the developed world, due to high standards of public hygiene, bacteria such as *E. coli* in local drinking-water supplies are far from unknown.

O Chlorine: this is the means by which bacteria have been eliminated from the Western world's water supply for over 100 years. While no one wants cholera and typhoid to resurface, chlorine brings its own problems, including an unpleasant taste and a tendency to react with other chemicals in the water to produce trihalomethanes (see below).

O Organic chemicals: many of these originate in pesticides and weedkillers or in factory and urban waste. As streams, rivers and lakes become contaminated, the chemicals find their way down into the water table and, from there, into our water supply. In Europe and the US there are set levels, above which organic chemicals are regarded as dangerous, although in the UK alone there were 36,000 reported water-pollution incidents in 1995. Even more worrying, new chemicals are being developed and put into use too quickly for their effects to be fully evaluated.

O Nitrate: usually traced to the extensive use of nitrate fertilizers or to sewage contamination, nitrate is not actually dangerous in drinking water until it reacts with other chemicals to form nitrite. If nitrate is converted into nitrite within the digestive tract, it may go on to form carcinogenic nitrosamines. Excessive levels of nitrate can also cause nitrate cyanosis, which is often called 'blue baby syndrome', in babies under six months. Nitrates are also found in food, particularly cured meats and intensively farmed vegetables.

O Trihalomethanes: these are powerful, poisonous compounds formed when chlorine reacts with dissolved organic chemicals (chloroform is a trihalomethane). They are carcinogenic and can damage cell structures in living organisms. *The American Journal of Public Health* estimates that about 9 per cent of bladder cancers and 15 per cent of rectal cancers are caused by the long-term consumption of drinking water that has been treated with chlorine.

O Polyaromatic hydrocarbons (PAHs): these originate mainly from the asphalt or bitumen coating placed on the inside of cast-iron or mild-steel pipelines to prevent corrosion. They are strongly suspected of being carcinogenic. The EC limit for PAHs in drinking water is 200 nanograms per $1^3/_4$ pints/1 litre, but readings of 4,000 nanograms have been found in Britain.

O Lead: although water usually leaves the water works with levels of heavy metals far below the permitted levels, by the time it reaches the consumer it often contains over five times the limit. Most lead in drinking water comes from old lead pipes or the lead solder used in joining newer pipes. Lead-contaminated water is a serious health threat, particularly to children and pregnant women. In children, problems range from learning difficulties and behavioural problems to mental and physical retardation. A study in *The Lancet* showed that children with a high level of lead in their blood scored on average 6 per cent lower in ability tests. In pregnant women, foetal growth and development may be affected. Adults with excessive amounts of lead in their systems can suffer from hypertension, strokes and heart disease. Lead accumulates in the body because there is no natural method of eliminating it and it can take 15–20 years before the effects become apparent. The problem is worse in soft-water areas (see below).

O Aluminium: this is the most bountiful metal on earth and it is used, as aluminium sulphate, as a form of water treatment in some water works. Where it occurs naturally it can be washed into the water table from surrounding rocks. There are clear links between high levels of aluminium and Alzheimer's disease. Aluminium also raises the acid content of water, leading to an increase of lead, cadmium and other metals that can be dissolved from pipework.

O Cadmium: this can be found in the water of houses with zinc-plated pipes. Like lead, it accumulates in the body and can cause stomach cramps, headaches, kidney failure and liver damage.

O Mercury: this is always removed at the water works. People who have a private well or spring, especially in an area of intensive farming, may however be at risk from mercury poisoning, which causes skin problems, mouth ulcers, loose teeth, internal bleeding, and liver and kidney damage.

O Fluoride: in many countries – such as Germany, Spain, France and Sweden – fluoridation of the water is illegal. In other countries fluoride is added to the water as a matter of course, in order to reduce tooth cavities. However, fluoride toxicity has been linked to genetic damage in plants and animals, to birth defects in humans (possibly including Down's syndrome) and to allergic reactions. There is also growing evidence that it can interfere with the metabolism of calcium, magnesium, manganese and vitamin C within the body.

O Medication: a growing concern is the level of painkillers, antibiotics and oestrogen (from the contraceptive pill) to be found in our water. Perhaps this is not so surprising when you consider that, in a city like London, the water you drink has already passed through 25 other people before it actually gets to you!

BOTTLED WATER

So is bottled water the only safe option? After all, have people not drunk bottled water for centuries because of its curative powers? Unfortunately, bottled water is not necessarily safer. Some bottled waters come from spas, but others consist simply of tap water that has been put through a filter to remove the taste of chlorine. Even the water that comes from a spa may have had to travel through polluted farmland and may have picked up chemicals en route.

Recently there have been a number of controversies concerning mineral water and casting doubt on its beneficial content. And, unlike tap water, which has to undergo 57 tests for possible contaminants, mineral water undergoes only 15 such tests. And European standards for factory-bottled water are actually lower than those for ordinary tap water.

Some of the added extras that have been found in mineral waters are exactly the same as those that scare us when they come out of the tap. Nitrates are found in some mineral waters; benzene, kerosene – even uranium – have been found in others. Doctors fear that excessive levels of calcium in mineral water may lead to the formation of kidney stones, while a high sodium content is believed to lead to high blood pressure.

Mineral water is not, however, the only water that is bottled. Spring and table waters are classified separately and require no tests whatsoever. However, like any water that comes out of the ground, spring water is all too likely to have been contaminated. This is all very confusing for the consumer, who simply wants to know what is safe to drink.

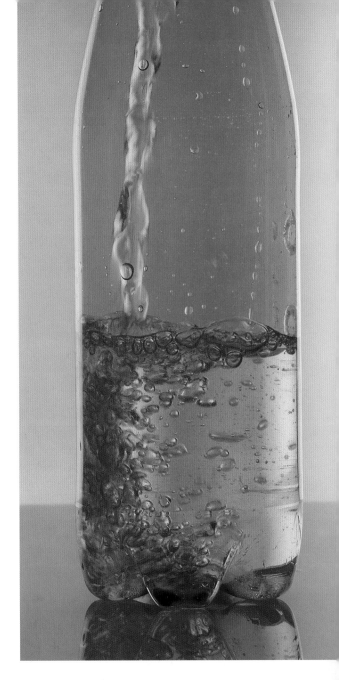

WATER WISDOM

Research by the US Environmental Studies Institute revealed that of 37 different brands of bottled water, 24 did not comply with the official standards.

FILTERED WATER

If tap water is more rigorously tested than bottled water, is there anything we can do to clean it up further? There are a few steps you can take to minimize the problems of contamination. Never use the hot tap for drinking water – hot water dissolves heavy metals into the water far more readily than cold. And always run the water for a minute or two first thing in the morning, so that you are drinking fresh from the mains, rather than water that has been collecting chemicals in the domestic pipes all night.

If you want to make even more of a difference, your best bet is to use a water filter. There are various types, from a simple jug on the kitchen counter to a water purifier for all your hot and cold water. Check carefully exactly what they promise to do. Some jug filters, for instance, may do nothing more than improve the taste of the chlorine, while others will reduce heavy metals – though only to a degree. For a more effective water treatment you need a filter that is attached to your water supply under the kitchen sink. A number of different processes may be used.

A carbon filter will reduce unpleasant odours and tastes, but will have no significant effect on heavy metals or bacteria. Reverse osmosis is the process by which water is forced, under pressure, through a semi-permeable membrane to leave behind many dissolved metals and virtually all bacteria, pesticides and insecticides. There are also water purifiers on the market that remove all these unwanted elements without sacrificing calcium and other important trace minerals that are actually beneficial to our health.

There are even whole-house water purifiers, which cleanse the bathing water as well as the drinking water. This may not be as sybaritic as it sounds. Skin absorption and inhalation from water are both currently being studied as a means of ingesting harmful chemicals. In fact, as long ago as 1984 findings published in *The American Journal of Public Health* revealed 63 per cent skin absorption of particular chemicals from water in a 15-minute period. Other studies have shown that showering in polluted water can result in very high rates of inhaled chemical absorption.

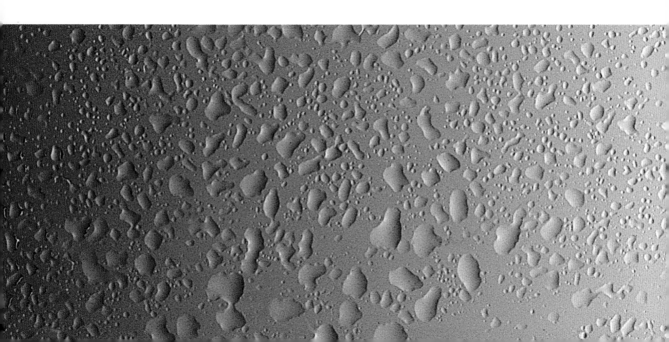

HARD AND SOFT WATER

You need to make sure that, whatever kind of filter you use, it gets rid of the undesirable chemicals and metals but retains the beneficial ones. Above all, do not get filters confused with water softeners. You do not want a water softener for your drinking water. While water softeners stop the kettle scaling up and make lathering more effective, soft water is much less healthy to drink than hard.

In spite of its name, soft water is actually more corrosive than hard, so it is much more likely to attack pipes and absorb their poisonous metals. Furthermore, the calcium and magnesium deposits in hard water appear to reduce the risks of heart attacks and strokes. The British Regional Heart Study analysed 253 towns from 1969 to 1973 and found 10–15 per cent fewer cardiovascular deaths in hard-water areas.

There is rather more controversy concerning sodium. While many doctors recommend a low-sodium diet for patients who are at risk from high blood pressure, other researchers dispute this, saying that it is the chloride (salt being sodium chloride), rather than the sodium, that causes the problem. Clearly, more research is needed into this subject but, in the meantime, if you use a water softener for your bathing water, make sure that you have another tap linked directly to the mains for your drinking water.

THE WATER ENERGIZER

Another form of research is currently investigating water purity. The Centre for Implosion Research in Plymouth has recently been looking at the bioenergetics of water in order to produce what is known as 'energized water'. Professor David Schweitzer examined water molecules through a fluorescent microscope with a magnification power of 4,000 to study the intensity and vibrancy of biophotons of clusters of H_2O molecules. Biophotons are molecular light emissions, which are thought to play a part in regulating cell growth and in the regeneration and control of biochemical processes. Ordinary tap water contains only a few scattered biophotons, whereas energized water has much more densely packed molecular clusters showing greatly increased biophoton emissions.

The energized water is produced using a process called implosion. This is the opposite of explosion – a suctional process that moves water in a powerful rhythmic, pulsating vortex. During implosion, the Centre for Implosion Research says, the water becomes highly energized with 'live' water, which is much more beneficial to our health than the water that travels through endless straight pipes on its way to our homes. In nature, of course, water only travels in a winding, snaking path, as can be seen in the route taken by rivers as they cut their way through the landscape.

Mains water pipes put increased pressure on our water, as well as bringing about greater friction and temperature changes, which – the Centre claims – all cause water to lose its energy.

The Centre has invented a spiralling copper device filled with this highly energized water, which can be used to recharge your existing water supply to the same high level. Studies have shown that by placing the device, known as the Vortex Water Energizer, next to ordinary 'lifeless' water, that water becomes energized, too. The energizer is placed on the main water-supply pipe and does not have to come directly into contact with the water itself. There is also a portable version, which the Centre says strengthens the immune system when carried in the pocket, by rebalancing the body's fluids; it can also be used to energize water, by placing the device next to a glass. This research is still in its infancy, but it will be interesting to follow developments over the next few years.

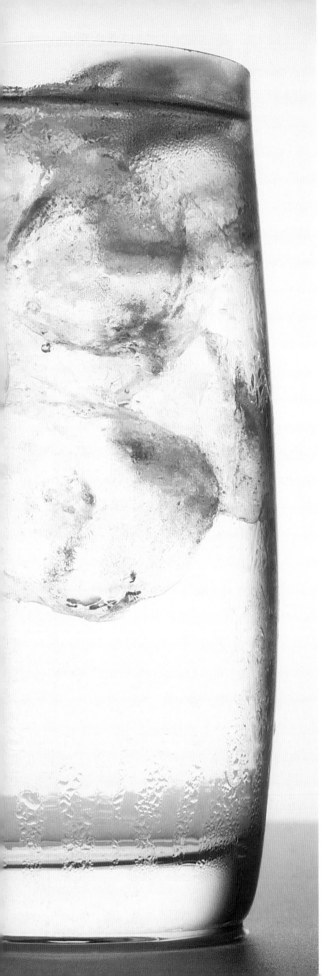

GETTING INTO HOT WATER

Most people automatically reach for a glass of ice-cold water to cool themselves down in hot weather. While this is indisputably refreshing, according to Ayurveda – or traditional Indian medicine – this is the very last thing you should do. In Ayurvedic medicine you are advised to drink only warm or room-temperature water, because cold and especially icy drinks douse the *agni,* or digestive power. The *agni* is so important because it is responsible for ridding the body of toxins, or *ama.* The stronger the *agni,* the more successful it is at flushing the *ama* from the body, preventing a build-up of impurities and consequent illness.

HERBAL TEAS

While drinking hot or warm water will be beneficial, many people find it rather boring. One solution is to add herbs. These not only improve the taste, but may also bring a wide variety of benefits, according to which herbs you use.

In this context 'herbal teas' – or, more correctly, infusions or tisanes – can include a great deal more (such as spices and fruit) than just herbs. One thing they certainly do not contain, however, is black tea, with its accompanying tannin and caffeine content. You can buy a wide variety of herbal infusions, either as loose mixtures or as teabags; you can also make your own with fresh herbs and spices.

When making an infusion, always use freshly boiled water and leave either the bought mixture or your own ingredients to infuse for much longer than you would ordinary black tea. This is especially true if you are using a root, such as ginger (when the drink is properly called a decoction rather than an infusion). Ginger needs to steep for at least 10 minutes in water before you drink it; or, better still, make up a whole flask and drink the decoction throughout the day and it will infuse increasingly hour by hour. Make sure that you chop the ginger up well first.

Below are some suggestions for herbal drinks, together with a note of their uses and beneficial side-effect (see page 130 for details on quantities). If you find a tea is too bitter, add a teaspoonful of organic honey to sweeten it.

SOOTHING HERBS

HERB	USES
Peppermint	A general pick-me-up; very good for soothing the digestion, relieving headache, mucus problems, morning sickness, travel sickness.
Ginger	Excellent for respiratory problems (colds, coughs, flu, sore throats), most digestive problems, poor circulation, fever, flatulence; a general stimulant.
Camomile	Very soothing, particularly to the nervous and digestive systems, but also on an emotional level; helps anxiety, headaches and insomnia; cystitis and water retention; good for children (with extra honey) to help them sleep, for colic and to soothe feverish illness.
Cinnamon/cloves/nutmeg	All three stimulate the digestive system; soothe fevers, colds, flu; promote good circulation.
Fennel	Very soothing for all digestive problems, morning sickness; good for children's stomach upsets (with honey) and for travel sickness.
Lemon balm	A soothing herb, good for calming and lifting the spirits (depression, nervous indigestion) and for insomnia.

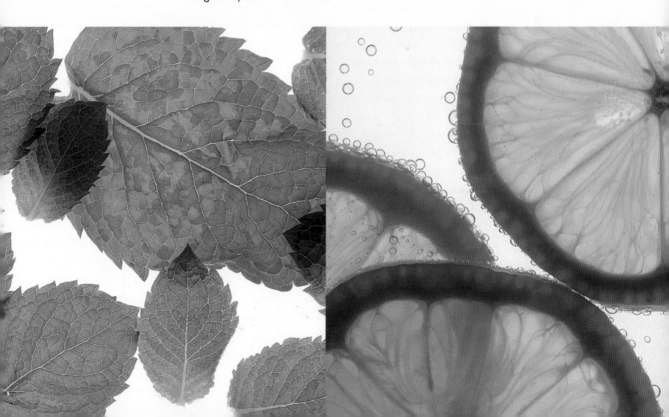

OTHER DRINKS

There are other drinks, both hot and cold, that can be beneficial *in addition to* your daily water quota. Your grandmother may well have told you that she fended off illness and looked after her complexion by drinking cabbage-water – the water left over after the cabbage had been cooked in it. In fact she was largely correct.

Many of the nutrients in vegetables disappear into the water during the cooking process, particularly if the vegetables are boiled for a long time. This is one reason why you should never overcook your vegetables – the longer you boil them, the more vital vitamins and other important trace elements are lost. However, as long as you do not put more than a pinch of salt (or, preferably, none at all) in the water, the liquid is worth drinking on its own. One of the most important elements in a deep detoxification programme is actually just a more complex version of Granny's cabbage-water. This vegetable broth is a cleansing and alkalizing hot drink, supplying masses of vitamins, minerals and trace elements. Even if you are not on a detox programme as such, vegetable broth is certainly worth taking, because it is such a beneficial drink. If you have one day a week – or even just one a month – when you drink only vegetable broth and eat just raw fruit and vegetables, this will have both a rehydrating and a deeply cleansing effect on your system. By the way, Granny was right on that other point, too – it does wonders for the complexion.

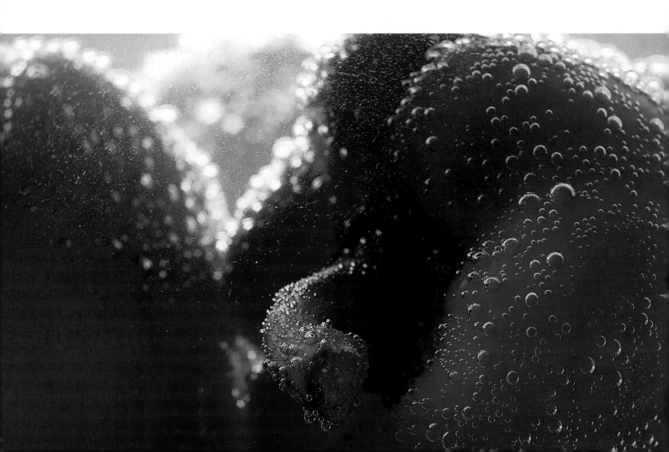

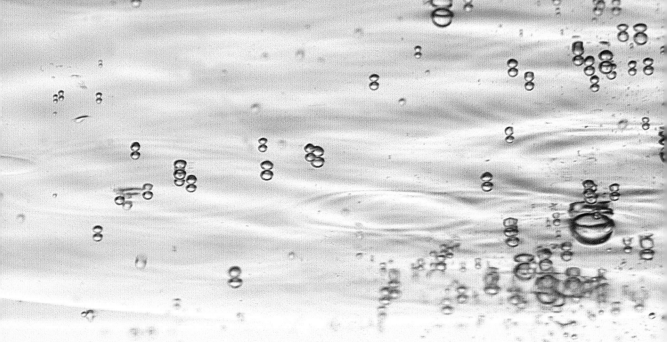

VEGETABLE BROTH

Use organic ingredients if you can get them and always clean the vegetables thoroughly, especially if they are not organic. There are vegetable bouillon powders that you can buy, but do read the list of ingredients carefully. In order to avoid additives, it is much better to make your own broth.

---

2 large potatoes

2 carrots

4 sticks of celery, with leaves

2 raw beetroot, with leaves

at least two other vegetables, including one green (e.g. cabbage, turnips, yams, broccoli, spinach, celeriac, leeks, onions, parsnip, spring greens, marrow, pumpkin)

3pt/1.75l still, bottled or filtered water

fresh herbs and spices, to taste (e.g. parsley, rosemary, ginger, chilli peppers, cayenne, coriander, thyme)

Wash or scrub all the vegetables thoroughly, but leave the peel on them, then chop roughly. Bring the water to the boil in a large, non-aluminium saucepan. Add the vegetables, herbs and spices quickly, leaving them for as little time as possible exposed to the air after chopping. Bring to the boil, cover and simmer for 45 minutes. Remove from the heat and allow to stand for a further 15 minutes. Strain the liquid into a clean pan and discard the vegetables. Drink the broth, one cup at a time, throughout the day, rewarming it in a saucepan *(not a microwave)* as necessary.

BODY BENEFITS

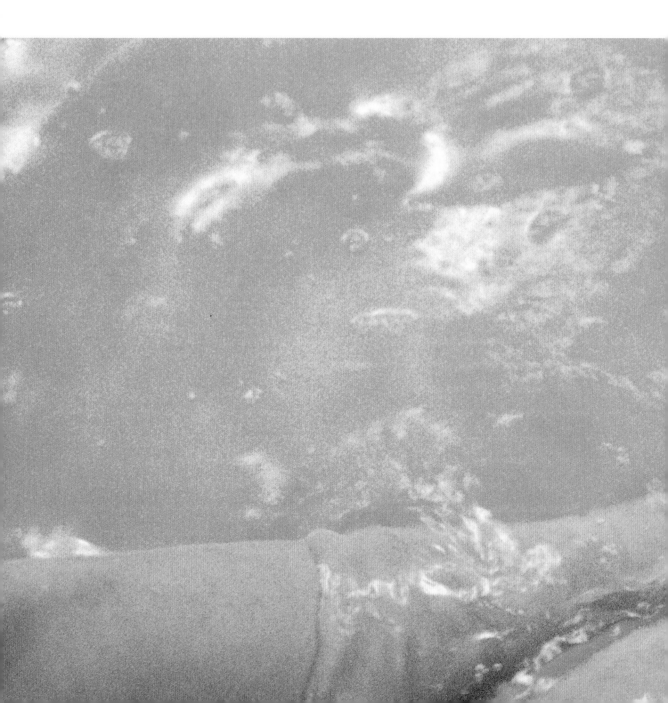

We now know that few of us drink sufficient quantities of water. This leaves most of us at least slightly dehydrated most of the time, in spite of the fact that chronic dehydration can exacerbate and even cause a host of diseases, including rheumatoid arthritis and ulcers. The benefits of rehydration are far-reaching: the digestive, eliminative, nervous and immune systems all function better; the skin improves, becoming softer and plumping out fine lines; we become more energetic and mentally alert. All this just by drinking a few more glasses of water every day? It really is that simple.

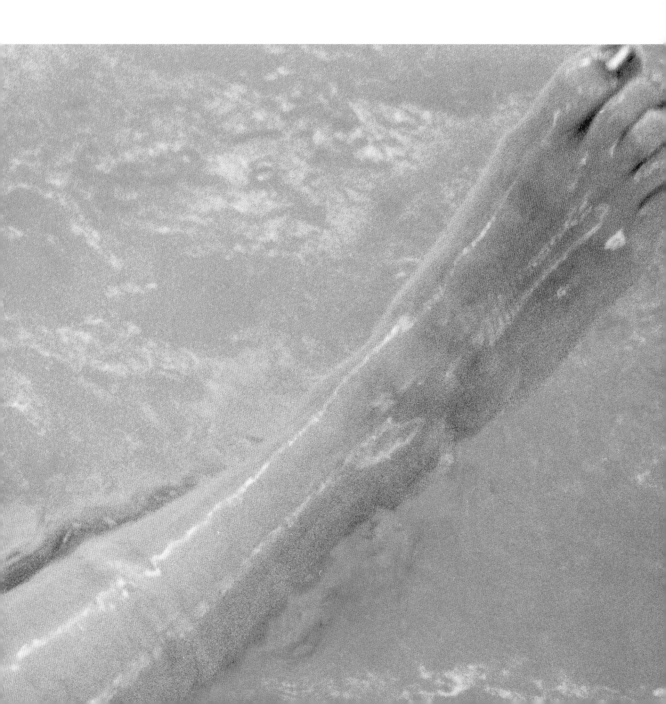

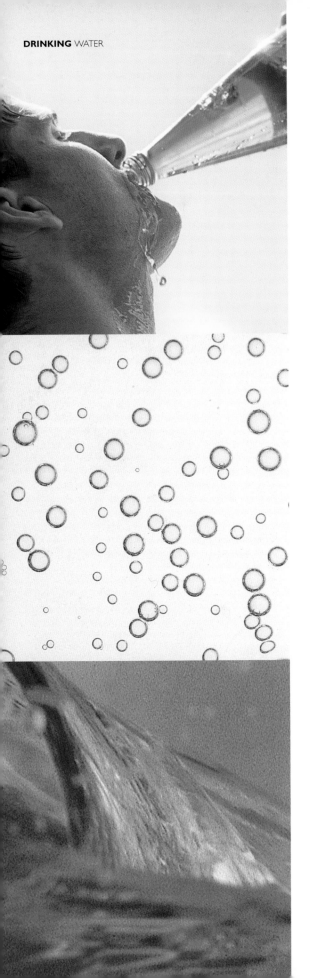

DEHYDRATION

Drinking enough water is beneficial to the whole body but there are particular organs and systems that suffer without it to such an extent that you soon become aware of a problem, even if you don't immediately recognize its cause. This is certainly true of the liver and the kidneys, those vital processors of the toxins that we take into our bodies on a daily basis.

THE LIVER

The liver is arguably the most hard-working organ of detoxification in the body. This is where the alcohol, caffeine, junk food, additives, drugs – the normal everyday poisons we consume – are neutralized. Once transformed by the liver into a form that will not cause the body harm, they are released back into the system for elimination.

However, if the liver has to work too hard – because we are consuming more toxins that it can possibly cope with – it has to store them and so the resulting backlog of waste builds up. The liver becomes increasingly sluggish and inefficient, toxins are not removed promptly and the body becomes susceptible to a whole range of illnesses from jaundice to headaches.

THE KIDNEYS

The kidneys are responsible for processing fluid wastes and purifying the bloodstream. They excrete toxins through the urine – and a change in the colour or smell of urine will often indicate a change in the state of the kidneys. As with the liver, if the kidneys are forced to work too hard because of an overload of toxins their function will inevitably deteriorate, leading to a wide variety of potential problems, such as kidney and bladder stones.

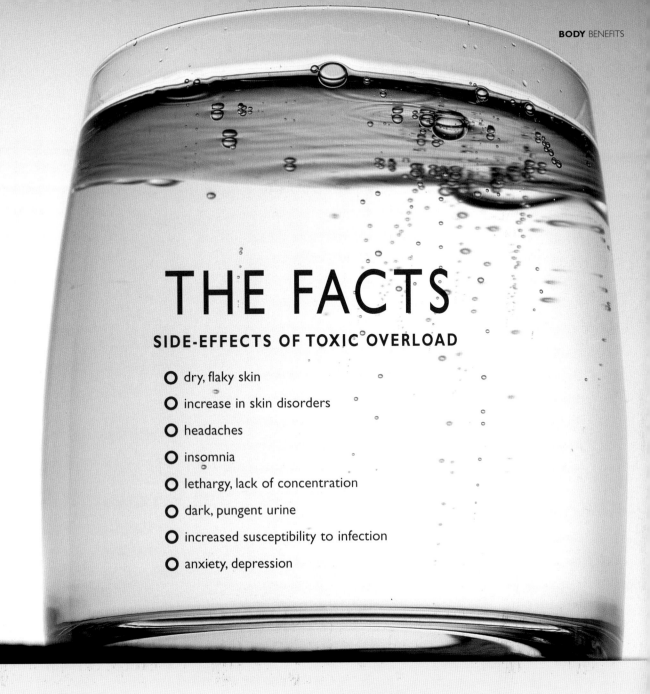

THE FACTS

SIDE-EFFECTS OF TOXIC OVERLOAD

- ○ dry, flaky skin
- ○ increase in skin disorders
- ○ headaches
- ○ insomnia
- ○ lethargy, lack of concentration
- ○ dark, pungent urine
- ○ increased susceptibility to infection
- ○ anxiety, depression

WATER WORKS

While a thorough detox is undoubtedly beneficial if the liver and kidneys have been under excessive pressure, drinking plenty of water will help to promote their normal function. Water increases the ability of the organs to process the waste by literally flushing it through. The more water you drink, the better they will work and, in doing so, the better you will look and feel.

Besides the more serious ailments mentioned, if your kidneys and liver are suffering from overwork and dehydration, there are a number of other side-effects you may experience, including those listed above.

For optimum results, you should drink water steadily throughout the day. This will keep a constant supply to the kidneys and liver and help with the neutralization of toxins and their elimination. When properly hydrated, many long-standing problems often miraculously disappear, including headaches, poor skin condition and a general feeling of being continually tired and below par.

THE DIGESTIVE SYSTEM

Food is the source of all our energy, and the healthier the food that we eat and the more efficiently we metabolize it, the healthier we will be in turn. Our food must pass through the digestive system, its nutrients being absorbed and waste products eliminated.

Unfortunately, the digestive system does not always function as efficiently as it should and, with too many toxins to dispose of and a poor diet to start with, it can become overworked, clogged up and consequently sluggish. Toxins build up and symptoms of disease appear – headaches, arthritis, constipation, irritable bowel syndrome or lowered immunity, to name but a few.

WASTE DISPOSAL

The colon, or large intestine, is the last stage in the digestive process and the place where many of the problems occur. It is a staggering 5ft/1.5m long and $2^{1}/_{2}$in/6cm in diameter and is populated by billions of friendly bacteria, which help to detoxify waste and guard against infection. The transit time from eating to a bowel movement should, if we are healthy, be around 24 hours. If, however, we are not healthy and have irregular or infrequent bowel movements, the colon can reabsorb the waste that should have left our bodies and pass it on to the bloodstream. This leads to a state known as autointoxication or, literally, self-poisoning.

Most of the underlying causes of autointoxication stem from a bad diet. Because we take into our bodies so many junk foods and drinks, alcohol, overprocessed food, too much fat, sugar and salt, medicines and drugs, cigarette smoke and atmospheric pollution, it is hardly surprising that, in the end, the body simply cannot cope.

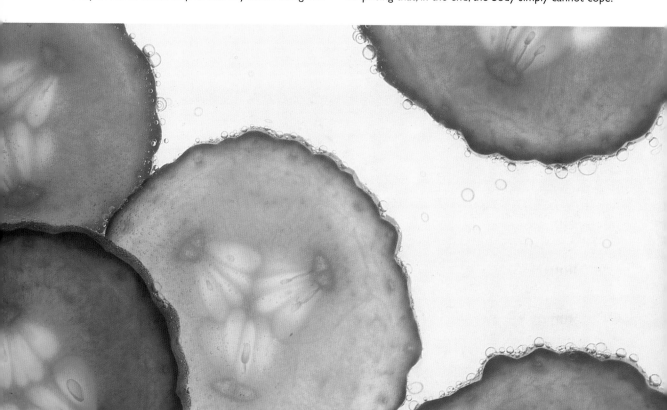

The digestive system needs to be given some help in order to run efficiently, and such assistance is easy enough to come by, even though most of us tend to ignore it. It is not that we do not eat enough, but that the food we are eating has lost much of its nutritional value through processing and is packed full of fat, sugar, salt and nutritionally worthless preservatives, colourings and flavourings. It is this very type of diet that is linked to heart disease and many other serious conditions.

THE RIGHT KIND OF FIBRE

The diet we should be eating is one that has a high proportion of fibre – fresh (preferably organic) fruit and vegetables (plenty of them raw), whole grains and lots of water. All of these encourage the rhythmical contraction of the intestinal walls, which is known as peristalsis, without which toxic effects are bound to ensue. Fibre in the form of fruit and vegetables is much kinder to the digestive tract than cereal 'roughage', which can irritate the intestine in some people. Fruit and vegetables also contain a great deal of water, and water is itself probably the single most important factor in the functioning of the intestine. Because the colon absorbs water from food in preparation for eliminating solids, the contents of the lower intestine can become very dry. The drier they become, the more likely they are to get stuck in the pockets (diverticuli) of the colon instead of being eliminated. So the more water we drink, the easier it is for waste to be moved along.

DRINKING IN BULK

There are a number of drinks with added bulk that help to force waste through the intestine. These are particularly useful if you suffer from constipation or other bowel problems, or if you are detoxifying. Of the bulking agents available, psyllium seeds are probably the most efficient and are readily available from health-food stores. As they pass through the gut, they expand to between 10 and 15 times their original size and push waste through the intestine. Add a teaspoonful of seeds to a large glass of water, after which you should drink at least two more large glasses of water.

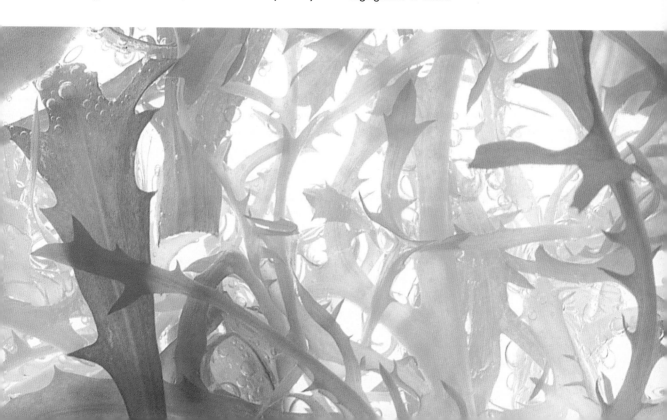

THE IMMUNE SYSTEM

When any of the major organs dealing with detoxification or elimination are stressed and overloaded, it is the immune system that is likely to suffer. Our bodies are profoundly complex organisms which, on a cellular level, are in a state of constant growth and renewal. Every day they rid themselves of old, damaged or dead cells and replace them with new, healthy ones.

The body has its own set of priorities for its metabolism. So, should we fall ill, our bodies concentrate on repelling invading infections and on the healing process. The organs of the body are prioritized, too – this is why, in extreme cold, the body will keep the vital organs working at the expense of the extremities (hence frostbite occurring first in the toes or fingers).

For most of us, illness and infection are, fortunately, only occasional problems and, once returned to a healthy state, the body can go back to its normal work of cleansing and renewal. However, the body reacts to a dehydrated, toxic state of health in much the same way as it does to disease. Instead of its everyday processes of cellular renewal, it focuses its energies on ridding itself of the toxins. And when the body is dehydrated, many of its organs and systems (in particular the kidneys, the digestive system and the lymphatic system) become sluggish and work below par.

THE LYMPHATIC SYSTEM

The lymphatic system resembles the circulation system, with the major difference that it does not have the heart to keep the fluid (lymph) moving. Instead, the lymph moves water, protein, white blood cells and electrolytes around the body as a result of the muscles contracting and relaxing. Keeping the lymph moving is vital because it plays such a central part in the health of the immune system. Essentially, it is the body's waste disposal – it gets rid of toxins and dead cells, particles of pollution and antibiotics. The lymphatic system breaks down these toxins and makes them safe before they pass back into the bloodstream, then on to either the liver or kidneys, or out of the body directly in the form of sweat.

The lymph channels lie just beneath the skin, and lymph itself is that clear fluid that seeps out when you graze or burn yourself. The lymph glands – in the neck, the armpits and the groin – often swell up during infection. The lymphocyte cells produced in these glands reach all the tissues of the body, where they form its principal defence against disease.

The greater the flow of lymph, the healthier the body, which is why water is so important to it. If the body becomes dehydrated, the lymph flow is weakened and we become less resistant to infection from outside and, indeed, from within – the body becoming less able to deal with its own damaged or diseased cells.

LIGHTENING THE LOAD

Drinking $3^{1}/_{2}$pints/2 litres of pure water every day is the simplest method of lightening the load on the lymphatic system. And by stimulating the lymphatic system, detoxification becomes more efficient, too.

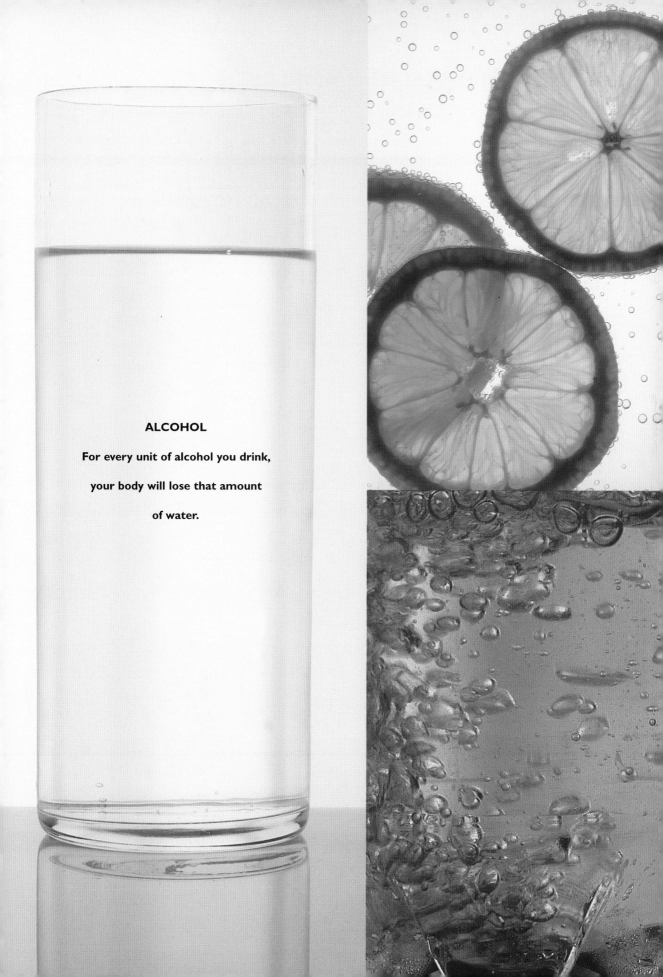

ALCOHOL

For every unit of alcohol you drink,

your body will lose that amount

of water.

STIMULATING THE LYMPHATIC SYSTEM

Unlike the circulation of the blood, the lymph has no pump to keep it moving. Given that the better the flow, the healthier it is, stimulating the lymph circulation is obviously vital. Drinking sufficient water, as we have just seen, is extremely important in stimulating the lymphatic system, but there are other ways to help the lymph towards optimum health.

MANUAL LYMPHATIC DRAINAGE

Manual lymph drainage (MLD) is a form of massage, which, by accelerating the workings of the lymphatic system, reduces many of the symptoms that are related to overstretching of the system. These include bloating, cellulite and PMS. However, MLD is also believed to be useful for accelerating the healing of burns and sprains and in cases of respiratory illness, such as bronchitis.

MLD is an extremely relaxing therapy and the very gentle strokes that are used are so unlike conventional massage that it may feel as if little is happening. However, with a properly qualified MLD therapist, this is a very effective way of stimulating the lymphatic system. Its adherents believe that it has two other useful side-effects. First, it is said to have a profoundly calming effect on the nervous system. Second, it is claimed that it can even be used as a beauty treatment. Particularly relevant here are skin problems, such as acne and scars, and any form of bloating, such as puffiness under the eyes.

The need for exercise

Lymphatic drainage is stimulated, too, by exercise. The exercise that works best for the lymphatic system is rhythmic (though not overvigorous) aerobic exercise. In fact, if you overstress the muscles, they actually produce more waste, which gives the lymphatic system even more work to do. Swimming is good therapy, as is rebounding – jumping on a mini-trampoline – for about 10–15 minutes. Both are particularly good because of their rhythmic quality, while rebounding's continual bouncing movement pushes the lymph cells into overdrive. Yoga and Chi Kung also stimulate the lymphatic system, amongst their other benefits.

Alternatively, one of the most easily available forms of suitable exercise is brisk walking, which is an excellent way of stimulating the lymph. The more pleasant the surroundings, the better. If you can, go to the country, the sea or a park. Wear loose, comfortable clothes and low-heeled shoes or trainers. Walk at a brisk pace, but do not feel that you have to run. Enjoy your surroundings, breathe deeply and spend at least an hour walking whenever you can – ideally two or three times a week.

On a daily basis, you can also include more walking in your routine. Get off the bus or tube a stop earlier when travelling to work and walk the extra distance. If you work in a high-rise block, take the stairs instead of the lift. Walk your children to school instead of driving them. There are lots of ways to incorporate walking into your life and, if it cuts down on exhaust fumes at the same time, you are helping with the airborne toxic overload, too!

SKIN BRUSHING

One of the other ways to stimulate the lymphatic system is by skin-brushing. If you do this on dry skin every day before you shower or bathe, it encourages lymph movement and helps to eliminate waste through the skin itself.

Skin-brushing (it is explained fully on pp. 82–3) is also probably one of the most useful weapons in the fight against cellulite. This is because it not only stimulates the lymphatic flow, it increases the blood circulation. At the same time, the texture of the skin itself is improved, becoming softer and smoother, so that the outer appearance of any cellulite improves, too.

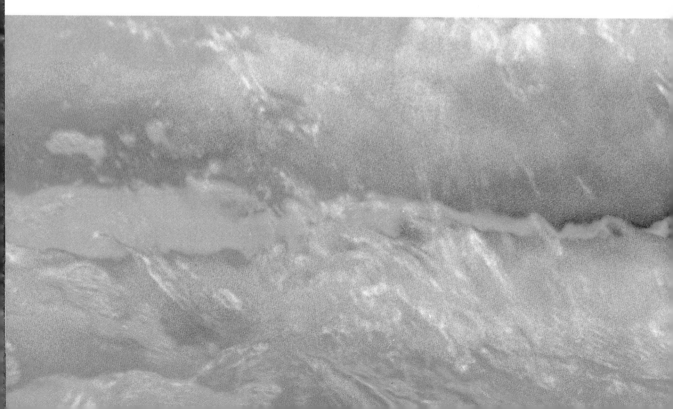

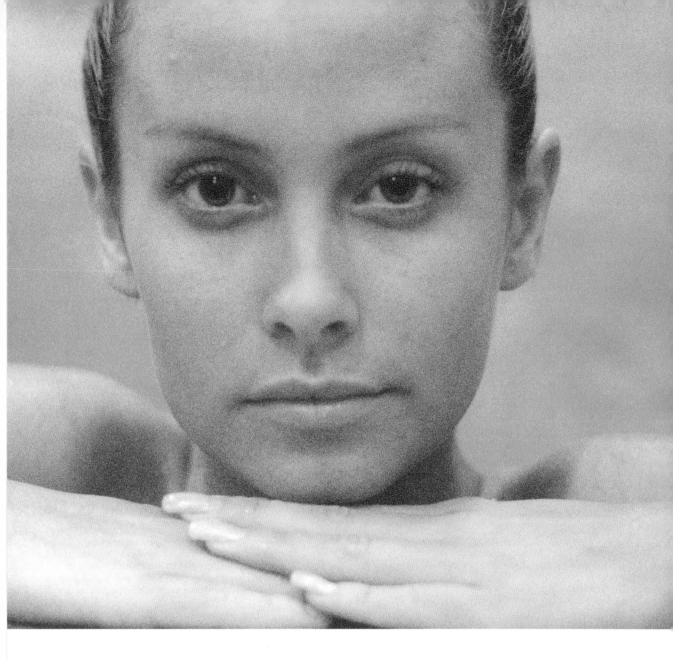

WATER'S BEAUTY BENEFITS

The hydration and toxicity levels of your body are nowhere more immediately obvious than in your skin. The skin is the largest organ of the body and it exhibits your state of health throughout your life. If you are tired, stressed or anxious, it will look pale; if your diet is poor or you have a hormonal imbalance, it will erupt into spots; if you sleep badly, it will look puffy. On the other hand, if you are healthy, your skin will bloom.

One of the most important ingredients for a healthy, glowing complexion is water. The beauty secret of young skin is that it holds 14 pints/8 litres of water, mostly buried in the dermis and hypodermis, the deeper layers of the skin. The epidermis (the topmost layer) contains less than 10 per cent of the skin's water content, but it is of course this layer – in the overall visible condition of your complexion – that reveals what lies beneath. It is not just that you *are* what you drink. It is that your skin *reflects* what you drink!

MOISTURE CONTENT

Dry skin is the most prone to the formation of fine lines and, eventually, to wrinkles. These form on the top layer, the epidermis, but the moisture content of the epidermis is fed from the dermis and hypodermis beneath. If these become dehydrated so that they cannot yield sufficient water to the epidermis, or if the movement of fluids around the body is inefficient and sluggish, the results will show in your complexion.

As we have seen, the body will be properly hydrated only if you drink around 3$^1/_2$ pints/2 litres of water daily. This will give the body a sufficiently high water content and will improve the functioning of all its organs and body systems. Exercise, too, is extremely valuable in activating all the bodily systems. It stimulates the circulation not only of the blood but also of the lymph and, as everyone knows, exercise gives the skin a healthy glow.

MOISTURE YIELD

One of the reasons that we need to keep replenishing our bodies with water is because we are losing it faster than is generally realized, because at the same time that the skin is being fed water from within, it is also rapidly yielding it to the atmosphere. Although most of us think of the skin as our outer protective layer, it is actually as leaky as a sieve. One of its functions, in fact, is to eliminate toxins from the body and, besides water, sweat contains uric acid, ammonia, urea and salts. These waste products can result in quite an unpleasant smell, especially if we are dehydrated, when they will exist in a more concentrated form. If the other principal organs of elimination are overworked – particularly the liver and kidneys – the skin has to work harder, too, to detoxify, often resulting in skin eruptions on the surface. The other function of sweat is to release cooling liquid on to hot skin, and so lower the temperature.

Sweating is, of course, most likely to happen when we are overheated and, if this happens because of exposure to the sun, we are, in effect, having to contend with a double whammy. The skin is losing its inner moisture and the sun's harmful rays are burning it and dehydrating it further – which in turn can lead to painful inflammation, premature ageing and skin cancer. Without sufficient water replenishment, the skin will inevitably suffer visibly. Whether the damage is in the form of an outbreak of spots or a dry, flaky or wrinkled complexion, dehydrated skin is at risk.

WATER WISDOM

The skin yields up to 3$^1/_2$ pints/1 litre of water to the atmosphere on a daily basis – hence the need to drink at least as much water again in response.

PROTECTING THE SKIN FROM WATER LOSS

While it is clearly vital to keep topping up with water so that our inner reserves of fluid remain high, there are other ways to help overall hydration levels by minimizing water loss from the skin itself.

In this particular endeavour some people start with an advantage. All skin contains an oil, known as sebum, which acts rather like a film to keep moisture in. The sebum of people with naturally oily skin is richer in the lipids that help 'seal' the skin than that of people with dry skin, and it therefore protects more effectively against moisture loss. But as we get older, our skin becomes drier, however oily it was to start with – which is why older skin is likely to become dry, scaly and lined.

PROTECTIVE OILS

The obvious way to give your skin protection is to feed it more oil and you can do this by applying oil in the form of moisturizer on a regular basis. Moisturizers are themselves a mixture of water and oil, and the amount that you need to moisturize depends on the dryness of your skin. You know your own skin better than anyone else. Its condition is likely to vary, according to the season and your diet, so its needs will change, too. If your skin is dry only some of the time, or only parts of it are dry, that is when and where you need to apply a moisturizer. On the other hand, if your skin is excessively dry all of the time, then you need to use a moisturizer constantly.

Today there are moisturizers that contain humectants, such as glycerine and hyaluronic acid, which absorb moisture from the atmosphere and pass it into your skin. Alpha hydroxy acids (AHAs) are another newly widespread ingredient in moisturizers and are thought to improve the skin's capacity to retain moisture.

The most important moisturizer for the complexion, however, is one that also contains a sunscreen. This will not only keep moisture in, but will also keep the sun's damaging rays out. For healthy skin, you should wear a sunscreen all year round and never sunbathe – the sun not only ages the skin, but can cause much more serious problems, including skin cancer. It can even, incidentally, suppress the functioning of the immune system. If you do get sunburnt, drink plenty of room-temperature water and apply a cold compress (see pp. 72–3) to any areas that are particularly inflamed.

REPLENISHING INNER OILS

You may also be able to improve the water-holding qualities of your skin by boosting its lipid production internally. More research is needed on this subject, but it is thought that raising your consumption of essential fatty acids (EFAs) will promote lipid production. EFAs are the fats that the body needs but cannot manufacture itself. You can buy EFAs in capsule form or introduce them to your diet by including foods in which they occur, such as oily fish (sardines, mackerel, tuna), seeds and nuts.

WATER WISDOM

Apply moisturiser to the body after a shower or bath while the skin is still damp. This helps it to hold on to the water on the skin's surface.

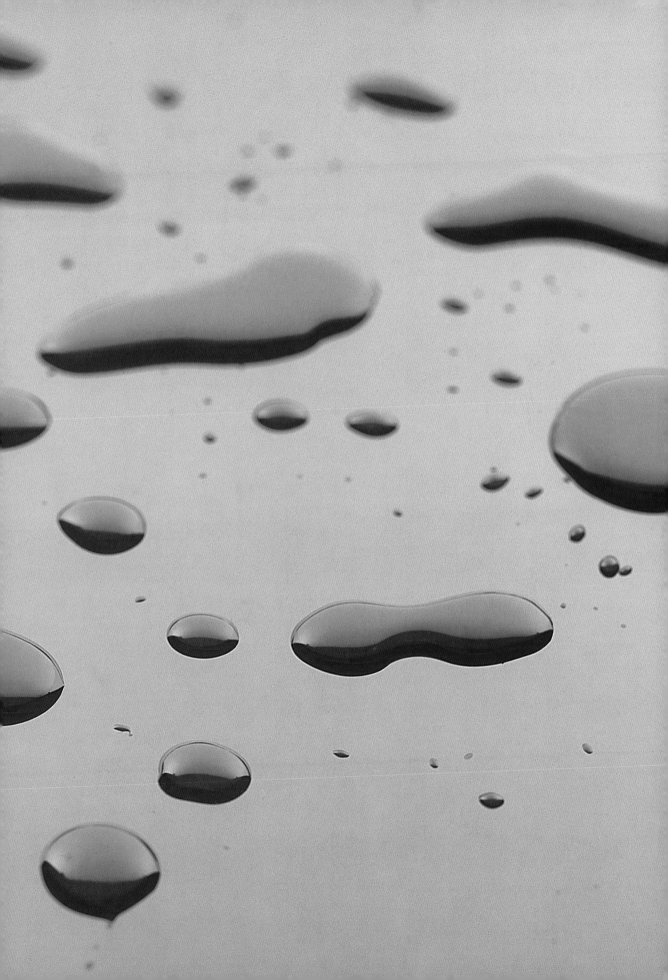

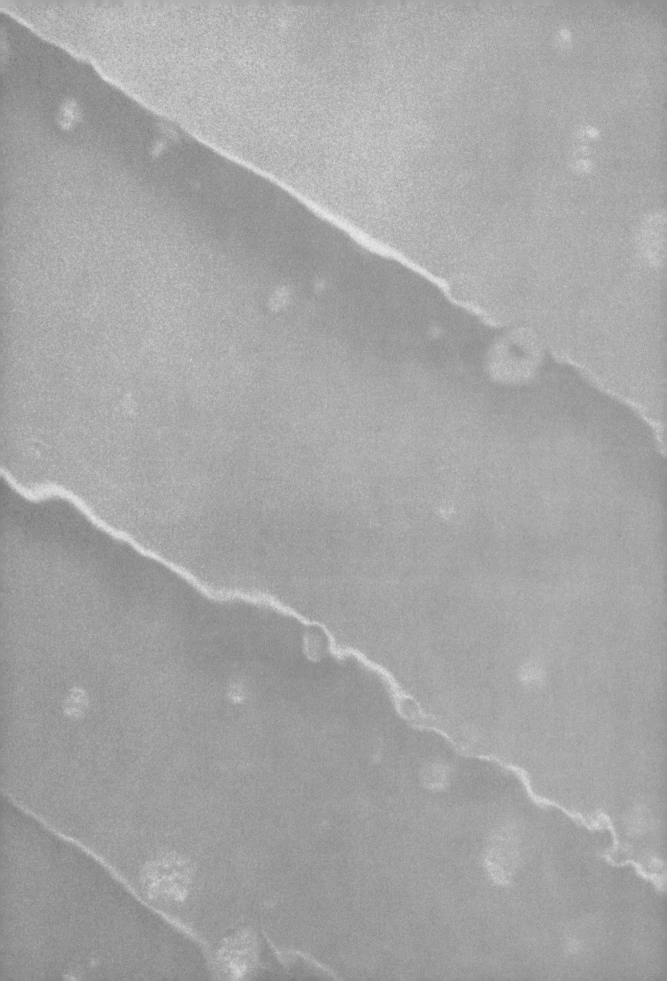

2 **WATER** THERAPIES

WATER PLEASURE

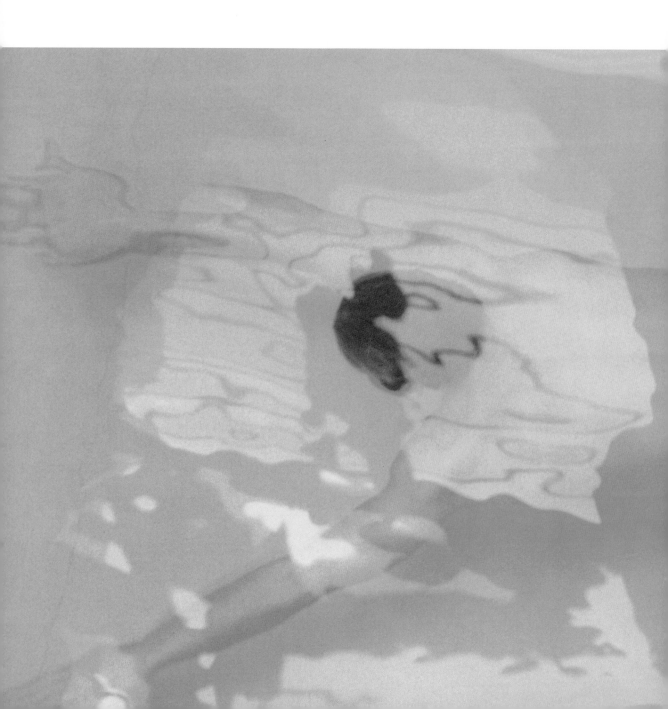

For a great many people holidays simply mean water. As children, we set off for the sea in the summer and wait with bated breath for that first thrilling glimpse of it. The days that follow are spent in it, on it or by it. And somehow the magic never flags, from that first day right to the last.

Perhaps it is the memory of that childhood magic that persists in later life and draws us back year after year to the sea. Perhaps it is because, beyond the conscious memory of humankind, an older primeval memory draws us back to our first watery home. Certainly we have devised every imaginable way of spending time in it or on it, whether in diving suits, sailing boats or on water-skis. We may swim in it all day, then return in the evening to walk along the water's edge, with the sea lapping at our ankles. Swimming with sea creatures, and in particular dolphins, has even become a form of emotional therapy for people who are seriously ill or for deeply disturbed children.

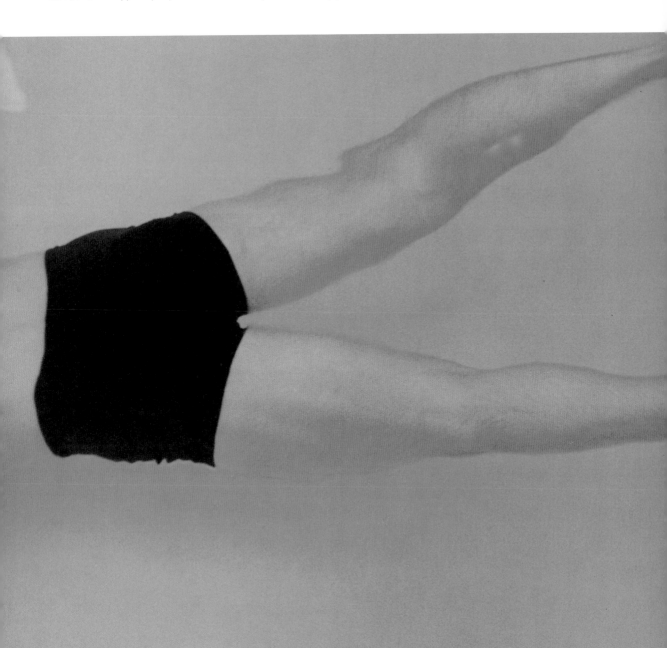

TOTAL IMMERSION

Simply being immersed in water has a simultaneously calming and uplifting effect on the mind. No doubt this is the reason that so many people find swimming or some other form of exercise in water the most appealing way to keep fit.

Water's other great benefit is its protective factor. Its unique buoyancy protects the body from injury while exercising. On land, if you are running or taking part in a vigorous aerobics class, various joints in the body (most notably the knees) will be sustaining regular shocks, which, in the long term, are often damaging. In water, your weight is borne for you – one of the reasons why water is probably the safest place for the seriously overweight to start an exercise regime.

But is immersion in *any* water good for you? Some water has immediate advantages. Sea water, for instance, is full of beneficial minerals and salts. Thalassotherapy – sea-water therapy – works on the basis that these minerals can penetrate the skin and enter the bloodstream. Thalassotherapy treatments are discussed in more detail on pp. 74–5, but it is important to note here that their success rests on using certain beneficial substances extracted from the sea in the form of salts, seaweed and minerals. These substances are taken from relatively unpolluted waters and often undergo a cleaning process before use, while the purity of the water being used in thalassotherapy centres is itself strictly monitored.

Although there is widespread concern to achieve higher standards of cleanliness in the sea water around our coastlines, in populous areas the sea is often badly polluted. This can cause health problems for swimmers – skin disorders and digestive upsets being the most common. For this reason, if you are swimming in the sea, try to establish whether it is an area where it is safe to do so.

POOLS AND SPAS

Most people, however, do not live by the sea and, except when they are on holiday, are more likely to swim in a town pool or at their local health club. The water quality in these can vary enormously, with the particular problem being over-chlorination. Too much chlorine can give you stinging red eyes and affect the skin (especially if it is sensitive), making it dry, red and patchy. Health clubs are now increasingly aware of this problem, and you should be able to find one where the pool water is only lightly chlorinated. Some health clubs also have sea-water pools, especially if they are located near the coast, and these are very pleasant to swim in, as well as being more buoyant than ordinary pools.

At a hydrotherapy spa, you will usually find either mineral water or hot spring water in which to swim and exercise. As with sea water, the minerals in these waters are believed to penetrate the bloodstream to create a wide variety of beneficial effects. Hydrotherapy spas generally have a particular speciality in terms of the treatments on offer. Many focus on specific ailments for which their water can bring relief – arthritis, rheumatism, skin conditions, circulation and weight problems, for instance, are all widely treated.

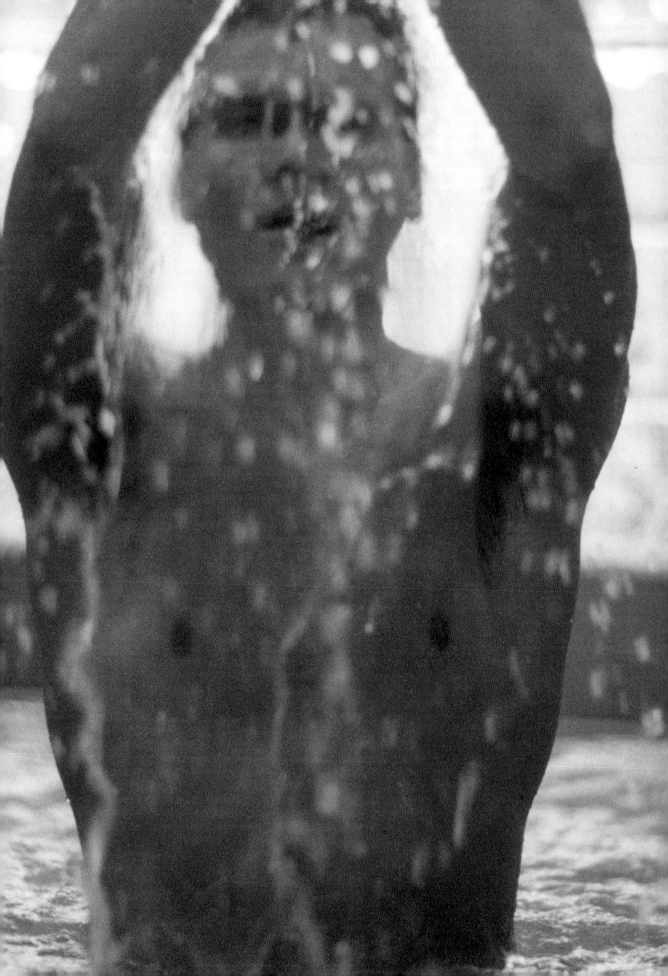

THE BENEFITS OF SWIMMING

Swimming is one of the most beneficial forms of aerobic exercise, as well as one of the safest. It is not a high-impact activity, like running, so many people who have sustained injuries (especially joint injuries) can swim safely without fear of causing further damage.

Swimming is a particularly beneficial form of exercise for anyone with stiff joints – whether from general lack of exercise or due to a specific condition, such as arthritis – because it often loosens up the problem areas without the risk of causing jerky (and hence potentially damaging) movements. For this reason, swimming is probably the best form of exercise for the elderly, who are particularly like to suffer from joint problems.

Water's natural resistance automatically increases the intensity of any movement you make, which means swimming is a very good way to tone muscles. If you have any areas of the body you particularly want to tone, combine swimming with some water aerobic exercises (see page 61). Simply walking the width of the pool a few times in shoulder-deep water is good for toning and, if brisk enough, as an aerobic exercise, too.

Drink plenty of water before you begin and after you have finished swimming. Just being in the water has the effect of stimulating kidney production by 700 per cent – which is why you always want to urinate when you get out of the pool!

ANTE-NATAL SWIMMING

Pregnant women form another group who benefit from regular swimming. Swimming is beneficial throughout pregnancy but, in the later months, it also has the psychological advantage of letting you feel weightless when most of the rest of the time you feel like a beached whale! Simply floating for a while for relaxation – in itself part of the preparation for childbirth – is a good way of finishing your swimming session. There is also a school of thought that claims that swimming is as enjoyable for the unborn child as it is for the mother, and many ante-natal classes in the pool include a gentle,

DIFFERENT SWIMMING STROKES

STROKE	AIM
Breaststroke	Tones the inner leg and upper arm muscles, but not recommended for anyone with neck, lumbar or other back problems, or for pregnant women.
Crawl	Excellent aerobic exercise. Good for toning the arm muscles and releasing stiff shoulder joints.
Backstroke	The gentlest stroke, particularly beneficial for the elderly, as it releases the shoulder joints; the best stroke for pregnant women.
Butterfly	The best aerobic exercise and stamina-builder, but only for those who are already fit.

self-administered abdominal massage. Swimming is good post-natal exercise, too. Relaxin, a hormone secreted during early pregnancy, which causes the mother's ligaments to stretch in order to make room for the baby, remains in the body for up to five months after the birth. During this period, joints and ligaments remain vulnerable, so high-impact exercise should be avoided, but swimming is a very good way to get back into shape.

SWIMMING FOR THE OVERWEIGHT

For anyone who is overweight, swimming is an extremely effective way to start an exercise programme and, indeed, to lose weight. Exercising on land can be particularly hazardous for anyone who is overweight, because most land exercise is, by definition, weight-bearing. The extra weight becomes an added strain on the joints, muscles and ligaments, predisposing them to injury. Swimming reduces these risks dramatically.

Of course, anyone overweight is also putting an extra strain on the heart when exercising, and care must be taken, especially if you are starting to exercise after a long break. Build up gradually and take it slowly at first. If you are seriously overweight, get medical advice before you start.

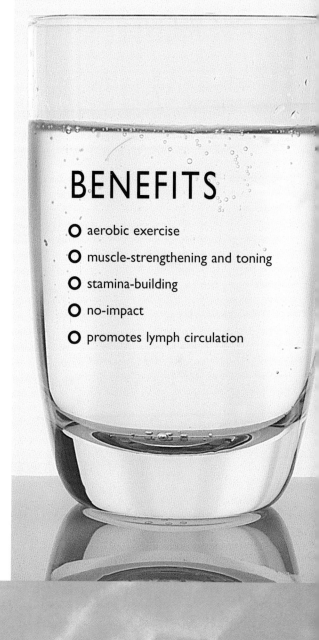

BENEFITS

- O aerobic exercise
- O muscle-strengthening and toning
- O stamina-building
- O no-impact
- O promotes lymph circulation

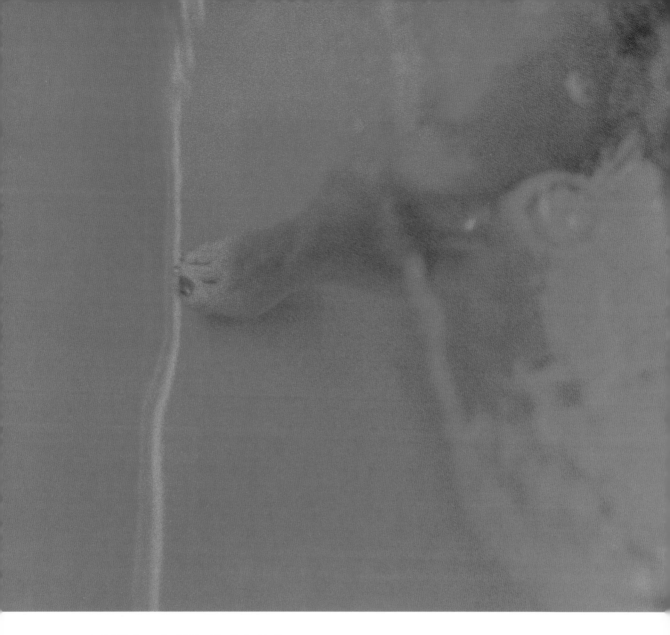

WATER AEROBICS

Water aerobics means, quite simply, exercising in water. It draws both on rehabilitative hydrotherapy techniques as well as on ordinary land-based forms of aerobic exercise. For the same reasons as swimming, it is a good way to get fit without the risk of injury. And, because you can also use the resistance of water almost as you would use weights or machines in a gym, it is excellent for targeting particular areas of the body that need toning.

There are water aerobics classes at most swimming pools and health clubs and they are often designed to fit particular needs – general fitness, toning, flexibility, ante-natal classes, over-50s classes – so you will usually be able to find one to suit you. As with any form of exercise, it is always best to have a teacher supervising you, at least to start with. Here, however, are some simple water aerobics movements to achieve specific results or to relieve particular problems.

WATER EXERCISES

EXERCISE	AIM	HOW TO DO IT
Arm lunges	For increased mobility of the neck, shoulders, lower back; an arm-toner.	Stand in the pool with the water at shoulder level, the feet hip-width apart, hands on hips. Take the right arm to shoulder height and reach across the body, bending the left leg up as you do so, to increase the stretch, and pushing the water away. Repeat, on alternating sides, 10 times.
Squats	Tones the legs and buttocks, mobilizes the spine; good ante-natal exercise.	Stand at the side of the pool, holding on to the edge, with the legs hip-width apart and the water chest-high. With the knees pointing outwards, bend them so that the tail of the spine drops straight down. Hold for a count of 10, then come up. Repeat 10 times.
Scissors	Tones the abdominals and buttocks.	Lie on top of the water, facing downwards and holding on to the side. Keeping the tummy in well and the legs under the water, scissor the legs up and down, as if you are taking giant-sized, straight-legged steps. Take a deep breath each time, before repeating 10 times.
Shoulder circles	Increases mobility of the neck and shoulders.	Stand feet slightly apart, with the water up to the neck, then slowly circle the shoulders forwards, upwards and back, 10 times. Then reverse the movement for another 10 repeats.
Press-ups	Strengthens the triceps and biceps.	Stand facing the side of the pool, with water up to the neck and the arms outstretched and holding on to the side. Keep the feet together and the legs straight. Flex the elbows so that the body moves in one piece towards the side of the pool, then straighten them again. Do 10 press-ups.
Leg swings	Improves mobility of the hips and lower back; tones the legs.	Stand at the side of the pool, with one hand resting on the edge. Keeping the knee facing forwards and the leg straight, swing the leg forward, then behind you, 10 times. Turn and repeat using the other leg.
Back leg swings	Tones the buttocks.	Facing the side, in chest-high water, lift one leg straight out to the side, keeping the knee facing forwards. Bring it back, then take it behind to cross the other leg. Repeat 10 times on each leg.

HYDROTHERAPY
TREATMENTS

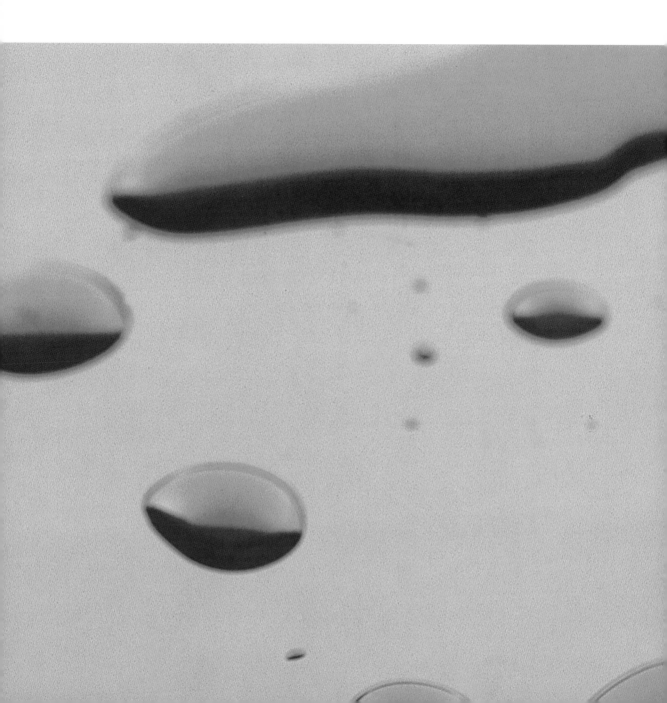

Although hydrotherapy was, until recently, almost forgotten in the UK and the United States, in Europe it has remained very much a part of mainstream health care. In Germany, France, Switzerland, Austria, Turkey, Russia and other eastern European countries there are a vast number of spas, as well as hydrotherapy departments in hospitals, all regarded as an important part of that country's national health service. Some of the treatments available are directed at specific – and sometimes serious – ailments, but there is, too, a great deal of preventative health care at the heart of hydrotherapy.

The power of water to heal, stimulate and relax is remarkable – and, for many people, surprising – but perhaps most remarkable of all is that, essentially, water treatment in all its forms is simply a means of helping the body to cure, cleanse or strengthen itself. This means that it is free of harmful side-effects.

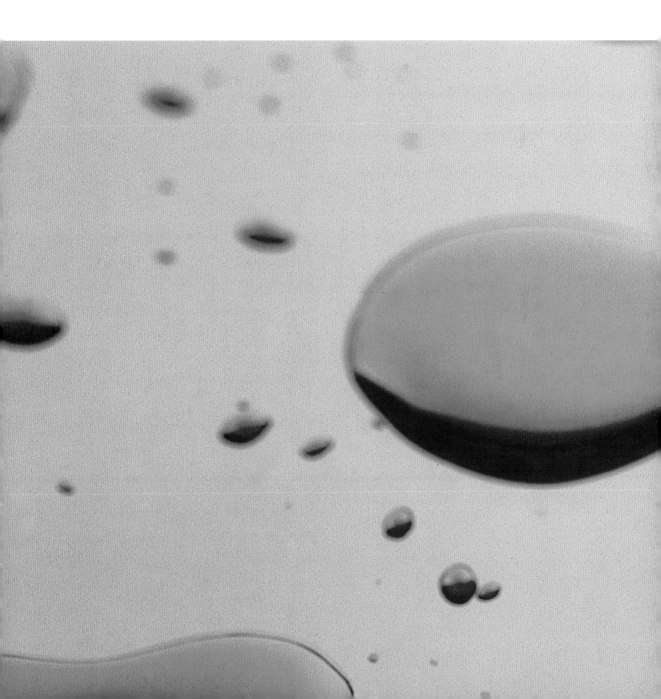

HOW HYDROTHERAPY WORKS

Fundamentally, hydrotherapy works by stimulating the body's own processes. Its underlying principles have remained unchanged for centuries but, in recent years, they have finally received the boost of scientific proof, and the physiological effects of hydrotherapy are now seen to be quite remarkable.

The psychological effects of hydrotherapy are also important – as we have seen, being in water promotes a sense of well-being and helps to relieve stress. Hydrotherapy treatments basically consist of applications to the body of hot and cold water. These include baths of numerous different kinds; compresses and wraps applied directly to the body; water massages; inhalations; and simple movements or exercises performed in water. It may be difficult to believe that such simple treatments could have a profound effect on the body, but medical evidence has now shown that that is exactly what they do.

RAISING THE TEMPERATURE

Hot treatments include saunas and steam baths, hot baths and showers, and hot compresses and wraps – all of which act on the body by raising its temperature. Almost two and a half millennia ago, the Greek physician Hippocrates observed patients in the grip of malarial fever and found that the fever itself could suppress other, secondary ailments. Fever therapy, as it is known in naturopathy, became a lynchpin of early holistic treatment because of its power in fighting off infection. Today this may seem a strange view, when suppressing fever is the target of a vast pharmaceutical industry.

While no one would dispute that suffering from a fever can be an uncomfortable experience, the body produces fever to mobilize its defences in order to fight infection.

Raising body temperature strengthens the body's immune function in a variety of ways. First, it increases the number and mobility of white cells and antibodies in the blood and these destroy unfriendly invaders as well as metabolic toxins. Second, some of these invading micro-organisms are unable to survive the rise in temperature that occurs during a fever. Third, fever stimulates other organs and immune functions, including the production of interferon, a naturally occurring defensive substance in the body. Finally, when the body sweats it eliminates toxins.

BOOSTING IMMUNITY

Naturopaths believe that you do not have to be ill to benefit from a rise in temperature. Heat treatments therefore mimic the effects of fever and, in doing so, stimulate the brain, the nervous system and the circulation of lymph and blood – and the immune-protecting white blood-cell count increases in just the same way as it does during a naturally occurring fever. Toxins are eliminated through sweating and heat causes the muscles to relax and the joints to loosen; in general, it has a profoundly relaxing effect on the mind, too.

Heat treatments are, however, a double-edged sword. While they can be immensely beneficial, too prolonged a heat treatment can be enervating, even exhausting. Nor are they advisable for the very young or the very old or, in some cases, for pregnant women.

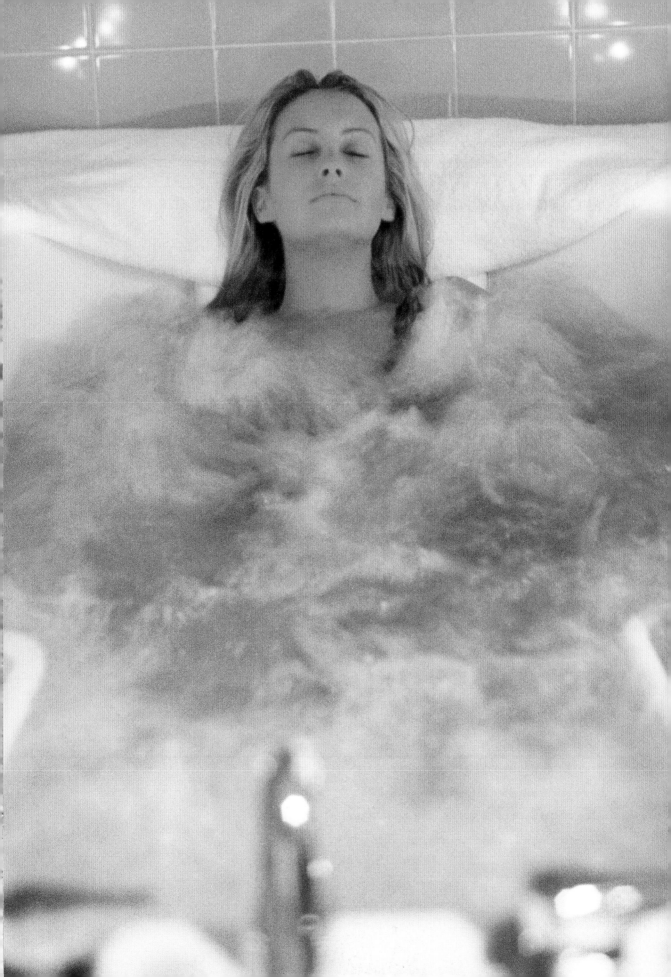

COLD TREATMENTS

Most hot treatments are regarded as a pleasurable activity in themselves, but can the same be said of cold treatments? In fact, as most cold treatments alternate with hot ones in hydrotherapy, these are not nearly as daunting as they might sound. Before you shudder, consider the benefits.

A short application of cold water has the immediate effect of slowing down the systems of the body and constricting the blood vessels. This is quickly followed by a surge of fresh, oxygen-enriched blood throughout the body, as the circulation increases and toxins are rapidly eliminated. One of the best-known uses of cold treatments is applying a cold pack to a surface bruise or inflammation so that the swelling and pain reduce.

Cold treatments include baths, showers, sitz baths, foot baths and local applications. They are usually of short duration, or used in alternation with hot applications, and are investigated in more detail below.

However, it is worth pointing out here that using short cold treatments on a regular basis has been shown to increase vitality and immunity, to the extent that people who take a daily quick cold shower are twice as immune to the common cold as those who do not.

ALTERNATING TREATMENTS

Alternating treatments are used extensively in hydrotherapy, and in the long term they are believed to build up a much higher general level of immunity. You can have alternating treatments in a variety of ways, some of which you can do at home, such as alternating hot and cold showers (see pp. 86–7). In a hydrotherapy spa, however, a great many more such treatments are on offer, and which ones you choose depends on whether you are relieving a specific problem or simply boosting your immune system and general health.

SITZ BATHS

Alternating baths are usually given in the form of sitz baths, though occasionally full bath treatments are given in hydrotherapy clinics for particular ailments. A sitz bath is, quite simply, one that you sit in (or, for many such treatments, two containers that you sit in alternately). Alternating sitz baths are used in many spas to treat gynaecological and bladder problems, constipation and haemorrhoids.

The sitz bath itself consists of two shallow containers, dividing the bath into two separate parts. One is filled with cold water, the other with hot. You begin by sitting in the hot side, with your feet in the cold. After about 3 minutes (depending on the problem and your own constitution), you change over so that your feet are in the hot water and you sit in the cold – this bit tends to necessitate a sharp intake of breath! Again, depending on your general state of health and the aim of the treatment, you can repeat the whole process up to 3 times, always ending by sitting in the cold water.

THE SCOTTISH DOUCHE

Another tried-and-tested alternating water treatment is the high-power hose, known as a *blitzguss* or Scottish douche. Immensely stimulating for the circulation, this

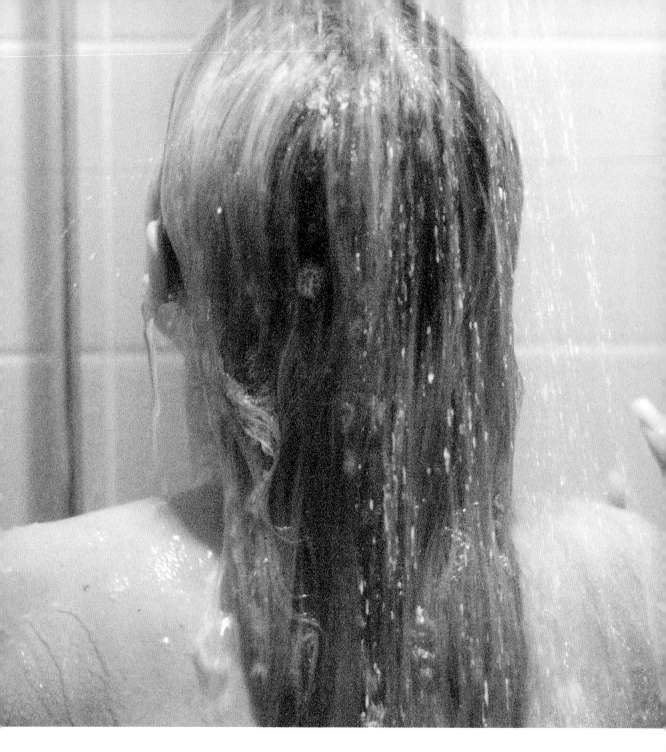

treatment is also powerfully cleansing and good for the skin. It takes place in a shower cubicle with side-bars for you to hang on to and is often preceded by a salt scrub (see pp. 84–5). Starting with a powerful jet of hot water, your back and the backs of your legs are hosed down for up to 3 minutes – and the jet is so strong that you really do need those side-bars. Then the water is turned to cold and you are hosed down in exactly the same way for a further minute. As with the alternating sitz baths, you can either finish at this point or repeat the process up to 3 times, always finishing with the cold water. After both types of treatment, you wrap up warmly in towels and rest for at least half an hour.

WATER MASSAGE

Massage is one of the most popular and pleasant therapies and there are a number of water treatments that incorporate massage to produce a deep relaxation of body and mind. There are mechanical massages, or water massage may be performed by a therapist.

Being submerged in water, especially warm water, makes the muscles relax and the joints soften, as well as bringing a state of tranquillity to the mind. The gentle massage of water in the form of underwater jets helps relieve stiffness and ease the pain of sprains, as well as being pleasantly relaxing and improving the circulation.

Jacuzzis are the most widespread form of underwater jet massages, but hydrotherapy baths are also on the increase. These are shaped like an ordinary bath but have two forms of water massage that alternate during treatment. One is a general water-jet massage, much like that of a jacuzzi, although as you are lying down it feels even more relaxing. The other is a more intense massage that begins at the feet and works its way slowly up the entire length of the body – sheer delight!

HYDROTHERM SPA MASSAGE

Another comparatively recent innovation is the hydrotherm spa massage system. Essentially, this consists of being massaged on a giant hot-water bottle – one of those ideas that is so simple you cannot understand why nobody came up with it before. The hydrotherm unit (or giant hot-water bottle) is the length of your torso, reaching up as far as your neck, while your head rests on a separate, unheated pillow for comfort.

You lie on your back throughout and allow the heat to penetrate your body, soothing any aches and pains and making the muscles relax. A therapist then gives you a massage – it is possible to do a very thorough back massage even though you are actually lying on your back – which is made doubly effective because of the heat penetrating the whole unit. The first time I tried this massage system, it felt a little strange, because the water was moving beneath me constantly. However, after a few minutes I relaxed into the feeling of being gently rocked on the water, and by the end of the session I had decided that this was the most profoundly relaxing massage I had ever experienced.

Hydrotherm spa massage is, incidentally, a boon for pregnant women, who often suffer from backache but, for obvious reasons, cannot have a normal massage, during which they would have to lie on their front. It is also a good way to experience a massage if you are underweight, fragile or elderly.

WATER TABLES

Another new trend is a massage table that turns into a water bed. I tried this out at the Zara Spa at the Dead Sea in Jordan. The water bed is incorporated as part of another treatment, such as a mud body wrap, and when you are wrapped in layers of mud, plastic and blankets, at the press of a button the massage table suddenly turns into a warm, supportive bath and you float in a state of deep relaxation.

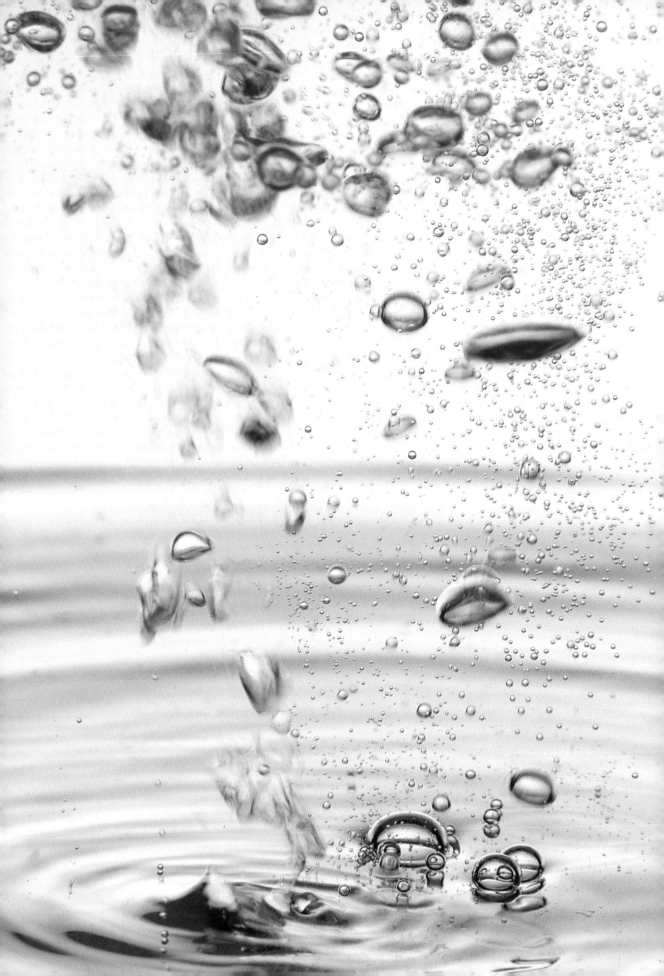

COMPRESSES, WRAPS AND SHEETS

Everyone is familiar with the idea of putting ice on an injury to dull the pain and bring down the swelling, and this is one common and everyday use of hydrotherapy.

If you do use an ice pack in this way, you should leave it on for a maximum of 10 minutes and always have a layer of damp towelling between you and the ice. I know of a case where someone gave herself frostbite by applying a freezer ice pack directly to her skin – not a pleasant experience!

A cold compress is safer than using ice next to the skin and, for many conditions – such as headaches, sprains, swollen joints or localized backache (see the Ailment Directory on pp. 98–9) – just as effective. If you are in a hydrotherapy spa, a cold compress may be used to treat a small area, or a pack may be used for a larger area or, indeed, the whole body. A pack comprises a cotton sheet, soaked in cold water and wrung out, then wrapped around you from the neck to the feet. Over this, a dry sheet or blanket is wrapped (there may be several layers of these) and you are then left to lie down for anything up to several hours. The initial stage,

of course, has a cooling effect on the body and is sometimes used alone in naturopathic medicine to relieve fevers. However, the body soon starts to generate heat and eventually sweats profusely, causing you to throw off toxins rapidly and, in the long term, build up your immunity and increase your vitality.

If the whole body is wrapped up in this way, it is called a whole body pack or Scottish mantle. There are also trunk packs (which reach from armpit to groin) and abdominal packs (from waist to groin), which have the same effects, although these are obviously concentrated on the wrapped area. They are also a more gentle introduction to this type of therapy than the full body wrap.

FOMENTATIONS

Fomentations use hot wet sheets or towels applied to the body. They are useful for congestion and muscular spasm (naturopaths recommend them for acute asthma attacks) and for period pains. You are wrapped in a dry sheet or blanket, just as you are with a pack, but fomentations are of much shorter duration. Each one is kept in place for only a few minutes, to be replaced by a freshly hot one. Fomentations can also be applied alternately – hot for up to 5 minutes, followed by cold for 1 minute – to stimulate the circulation of blood and lymph, as well as for back pain or bronchitis.

All of these treatments work on a deep level and should only be tried in a hydrotherapy spa, where they are always followed by a rest period of at least 30 minutes.

WATER WISDOM

Agriculture and industry are the greatest water consumers, although it is usually the residential consumers who are asked to make cuts.

THALASSOTHERAPY

Thalassotherapy is a form of hydrotherapy that uses sea water or other sea substances – notably minerals, seaweed, mud extracted from the sea and sand. It is particularly popular in France, Germany, Italy, Russia and, most famously of all, around the Dead Sea.

Thalassotherapy is beneficial for a number of ailments, including respiratory, circulatory and skin disorders, joint problems, rheumatism and arthritis. At Israel's Soroka Hospital on the Dead Sea, medical research has shown that arthritis patients who undergo courses of mud baths and packs generally register a marked improvement in such symptoms as stiffness, swollen fingers and restricted movement.

However, Dead Sea mud and salts are not only used as treatments for specific ailments. They are often used by therapists, too, in the form of body wraps, scrubs and baths. They contain a rich concentration of magnesium chloride, potassium chloride and bromine. At the Zara Spa on the Jordanian side of the Dead Sea, they use Dead Sea water for flotation pools, whirl pools, foot treading pools and various forms of massage jets. Special Dead Sea mud wraps are used to stimulate circulation and nourish the skin, and a Dead Sea salt scrub is a stimulating start to other treatments.

As a general boost to health, thalassotherapy is believed to encourage detoxification and increase immunity, stimulate the circulation of blood and lymph, soothe and help tone muscles and improve skin tone. Seaweed treatments, in particular, are thought to be useful in weight-loss programmes, as they speed up the elimination of toxins within the body and generally stimulate its functions. Besides mud and seaweed wraps, thalassotherapy also uses many of the methods already mentioned in this chapter, substituting sea water for ordinary water. It may involve exercise in sea water or simply immersion in it, so that the body can absorb the beneficial minerals.

Once purified, you can also drink the water, just as you drink mineral water in a hydrotherapy spa. The water of the Dead Sea, for instance, contains very high levels of the mineral selenium. Selenium is a potent anti-oxidant, a scavenger for free radicals – electrochemically unbalanced molecules, which are generated within our bodies as a result of stress and toxic overload and are responsible for a great deal of cellular destruction and disease. Together with vitamins A, C and E, selenium fights off free radicals and boosts health and general immunity. So far, you can only drink Dead Sea water at the Dead Sea itself. However, some of the mud and seaweed treatments are available for home use (see pp. 92–3).

WATER WISDOM

The Dead Sea is ten times saltier than the Mediterranean. Every 1³/₄ pints/1 litre of Dead Sea water contains 2¹/₂lb/1.25kg of salt and minerals.

DEAD SEA MINERALS

The waters of the Dead Sea contain an extraordinary cocktail of minerals: around 21 altogether, the most important ones being:

Calcium	Important for bone and teeth health, particularly in the elderly. It also helps to regulate the heart and nervous system.
Potassium	Vital for regulating the body's water balance, for muscular and nervous health. It is also used in cell metabolism.
Sodium	Regulates bodily fluids and blood pressure, although too much sodium is generally consumed in a high-salt Western diet.
Magnesium	Important for cellular health. It helps the body to metabolize sodium, potassium and calcium.
Bromides	Improve cellular repair and metabolism.
Iodine	Important for thyroid health and cell metabolism.
Sulphur	A potent detoxifier, essential for brain and liver metabolic processes and for strong hair and nails.

FLOTATION TANKS

Floating may seem an odd sort of therapy, and I must admit that it seemed to me unlikely to yield many benefits – until I actually tried it.

I thought it would be too claustrophobic to be relaxing, which is its principal aim (especially with the lights turned off). In fact, after about 15 minutes I found myself totally at ease in my watery environment, turned out the lights and floated contentedly for the rest of my allotted hour.

Unless you happen to be an astronaut, floating in water is the only time that your body is going to be free of the forces of gravity and this in itself is a quite extraordinary feeling. The combination of weightlessness and the absence of external stimuli enables the body to relax deeply – I experienced an almost instant release of tension in the small of my back, which I did not even know I was suffering from. External stimuli – gravity, temperature, touch, sight, sound – account for 90 per cent of normal neuro-muscular activity. When they are absent, even for an hour, the brain and the rest of the nervous system can achieve a state that is not only relaxing but, it is believed, rebalancing. Activity in the left, logical side of the brain is reduced, while activity in the right, creative side increases. Adherents of floating believe that this is one of the few times when your brain is in a state of harmony and that this helps you tap into a huge source of creativity and problem-solving.

PHYSICAL EFFECTS OF FLOATING

There are physical benefits to be had from floating, too. Because floating causes the muscles to relax so profoundly and the body to release endorphins (your body's own painkillers), it is a powerful aid to pain relief.

It is particularly beneficial for back pain, arthritis and migraine. By relieving the stresses of gravity, floating takes the weight off strained bones, joints and muscles, as well as increasing the efficiency of the blood circulation, and this in turn speeds up recovery after injury or physical exercise. What normally takes a long period of time – say, several days to recover after running a marathon – can be compressed into a matter of hours. This has made floating popular among professional sportsmen and -women.

Like other forms of profound relaxation, floating lowers the blood pressure and heart rate. And, because of the salts added to the water, it is even beneficial to the skin.

IN THE TANK

There are 700lb/320kg of Epsom salts added to 170 gallons/775 litres of water, and these are what make you so buoyant and give the water in a flotation tank its silky feel. Within the tank the water level is only around 10in/25cm deep and the water itself is heated to 93.5°F/34°C, which is skin temperature. There is a light within the tank and you may, of course, leave this on if you wish. However, there is quite a lot of space above you and the environment felt so relaxing that I floated in the dark.

Music is often played for the first 10 minutes while you relax, but for most of the time you are surrounded by silence. Audio-tape programmes for weight loss or to help overcome addictions such as smoking may be used in conjunction with flotation tanks to great effect.

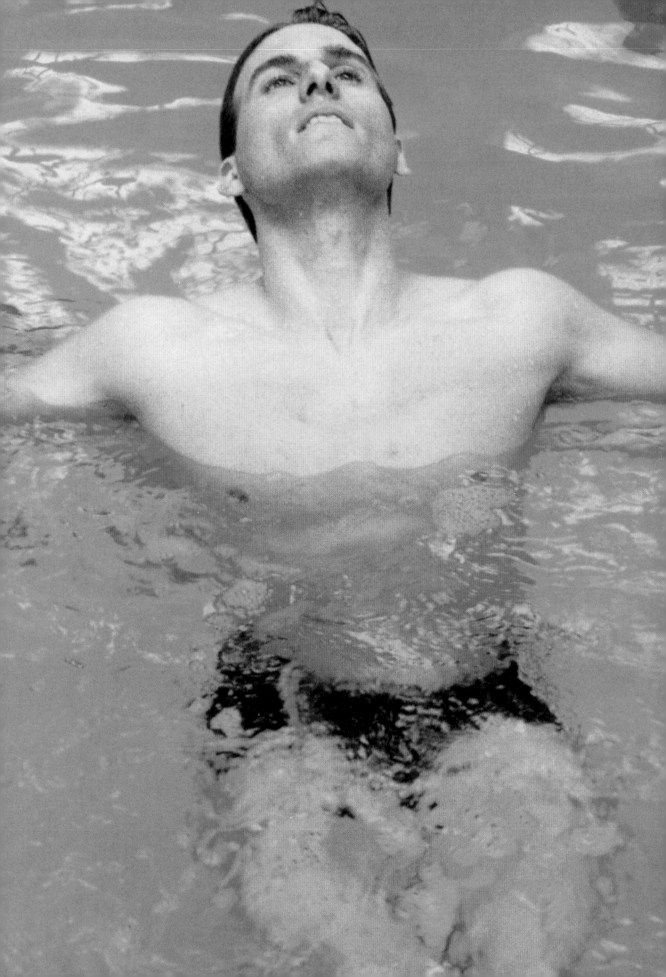

HYDROTHERAPY AT HOME

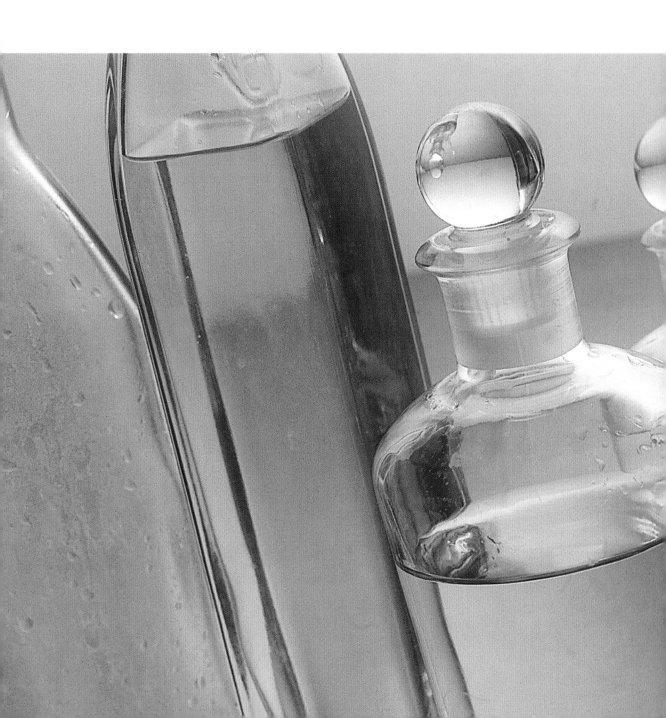

Going to a hydrotherapy or thalassotherapy spa is one of the most delightful ways to give yourself a health boost. However, this is something that can, at best, only be an occasional treat. Fortunately, there are numerous hydrotherapy treatments that you can do in your own home. Done on a regular basis, these will have a cumulatively beneficial effect on your health in general, and on your skin and immune system in particular.

If you are going to make your own hydrotherapy spa, there are a few points to bear in mind. First, while any bathroom that has a bath and shower will do, the more powerful the water pressure, the better the shower treatments will be. Second, you should make your bathroom as comfortable as possible. Make sure it is warm, and get a supply of large, absorbent towels – the fluffier, the better. These are powerful treatments and you will need to rest after each of them, for anything between a few minutes and half an hour.

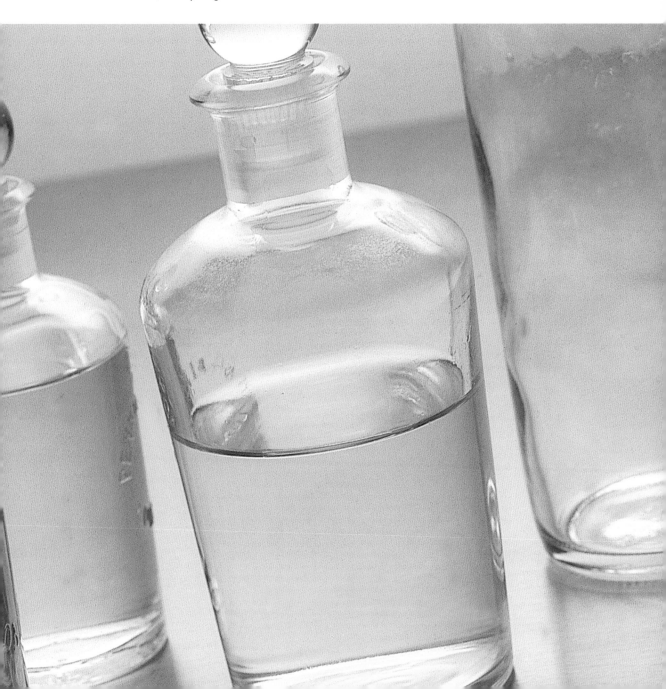

WATER ON THE FACE

Water is in itself a beauty treatment – we have seen that drinking enough pure water gives the skin a unique bloom. But, contrary to long-standing belief, water used on the face is also one of the best forms of cleanser. Until recently many people did not want to wash with water because they felt that their facial skin would suffer; that soap and water were too harsh for such a delicate area; and that cream- or oil-based cleansers would be both more gentle and more restorative of the protective oils within the skin.

In fact, most dermatologists now recommend using a cleanser that is washed away with water. There are several reasons for this. First, water soothes and rehydrates the skin. Second, water does not pull the skin around (unlike wiping off residue with a tissue or cotton wool). Third, it does remove all the dirt and oil (wipe-off cleansers often do not), providing that the soap or cleanser you use is suitable. A splash of cold water all over the face at the end of cleansing, both night and morning, is better than an expensive toner, too.

SOAP OR CLEANSER?

Of course, you do need to use something in combination with the water. Ordinary soap does a good enough job at cleansing, but it can dry out many skin types, as it washes away the skin's own oils and lipids. This is not much of a problem if you have oily skin, but if you have dry, sensitive or even combination skin you will effectively be removing the skin's protective layer. Soap that has added glycerine will have a less drying

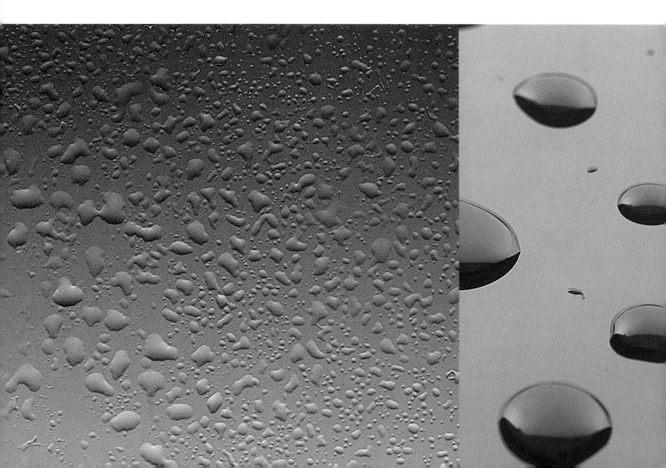

effect, but non-soap bars are likely to be just as drying for delicate skins. Liquid cleansers or gels that are washed off with water are extremely kind to sensitive skin as well as being efficient at cleansing.

EXFOLIATORS

Although toners are not really necessary if you clean your face with a water-based cleanser, exfoliating – the removal of dead skin cells from the surface – is essential. Whether you have oily skin (in which case exfoliating will keep down spot production) or dry skin (which will go dull or flaky without it), you should exfoliate once a week. Many cosmetic companies recommend more frequent exfoliation, especially if you have oily skin, but this, too, can lead to the removal of your skin's protective layer.

There are any number of exfoliators on the market, but, unless you particularly like the smell or texture of any

given product, it is not really necessary to buy one – instead you can use ordinary household salt (see p. 111 for how to carry out your own facial scrub and massage).

MOISTURIZERS

Cleansing the skin is the most important part of any skincare routine, but this is closely followed by protection. As you get older, the skin naturally becomes drier and you will need to moisturize more – although, of course, only on dry rather than oily areas. Moisturizer helps seal in the skin's own water content and, as you now know, the more you drink, the more this will be replenished.

Moisturizers are particularly useful at night when the skin can absorb them without any external daytime stresses. During the day, the best thing you can do for your skin is to wear a high-factor sun-protection cream (see p. 50).

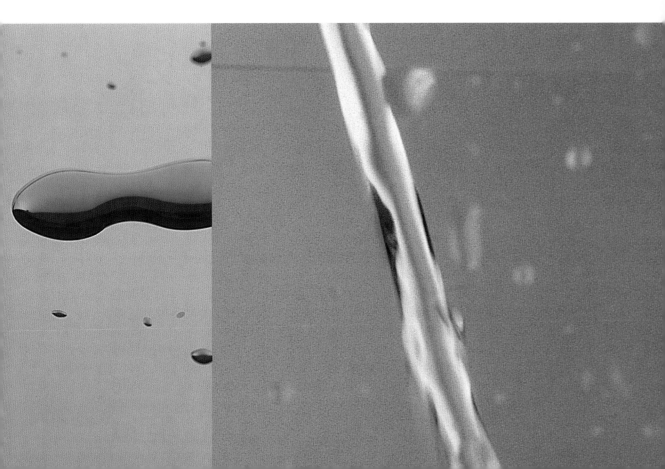

SKIN BRUSHING

As with so many hydrotherapy treatments, the combined effect of skin-brushing and alternating showers (see pp. 86–7) is to jump-start the system, stimulating the circulation of both the blood and the lymph. This, in turn, helps the body to slough off toxins more quickly and efficiently. It also makes the skin glow by removing the top dead, dull layer to reveal the fresher, smoother skin beneath. Combined with an increase in your water intake, this treatment will also have a highly beneficial effect on any areas of cellulite.

The technique is a simple one and you need only a body brush with natural bristles. There are various types of brush, all widely available at pharmacies and health-food stores and all quite appropriate, providing they are made from natural fibres – if in doubt, check with the sales assistant that it is natural and not a synthetic body brush.

You need to buy a body brush with a handle so that you will be able to reach your back. Some have detachable handles which you can remove while you brush your ams, legs and the front of your body. Alternatively, buy one mounted on long straps, which is ideal for using on the back and buttocks. At first, you may find the sensation quite rough, but after a few sessions most people find they get used to it and it feels exhilarating instead. When you first start, use a light pressure and only make it firmer as you become accustomed to it.

If after persevering for several sessions you still find the bristles too hard on your skin, you could try using raw silk gloves instead (see Resources on p. 141). These are worn on the hands like mitts and, although their surface is smoother than that of the brushes, they have an equally stimulating effect. Never brush skin that is inflamed or if you have any cuts, bruises or rashes.

Brushing the whole body will not take long: about 3–5 minutes. The important thing is to keep a steady rhythm going. If you do skin-brushing on a daily basis, you will see a real improvement in your skin's texture (it tends to get very soft), it will look more toned and slim, and it will also develop a healthy, rosy glow.

WATER WISDOM

Cellulite – which consists of trapped pockets of water, fat and toxins – is best dispersed by plenty of water plus skin brushing.

HOW TO SKIN-BRUSH

Skin-brushing is always done on dry skin. Make sure that the bathroom is warm and that you have plenty of towels to hand for when you get out of the shower.

Undress and sit on a chair or the edge of the bath so that you can easily reach your feet and lower legs. Take the brush, or put on the mitts, and begin with the sole of the right foot. If you are using a brush, use firm, rhythmic strokes to cover the sole several times. If you are using the mitts, you can make the movement more continuous, letting one hand follow the other. Continue the movement as seamlessly as possible over the top of the foot, up towards the ankle and on to the lower leg, making sure that you cover the whole surface – shin and calf. Always brush in an upwards direction.

Stand up and brush the area from the knee to the top of the thigh. Again, make sure that you cover the whole area several times with long, rhythmic, upward strokes. Continue brushing over the buttock, up as high as the waist. Now repeat the whole process on the left leg, starting again with the sole of the foot.

From the top of your buttocks, and keeping the movement in an upward direction, brush the whole of the back several times all the way up to the shoulders. This is the hardest area to cover completely – just reach as best you can.

Next, brush the right arm. Start with the palm of the hand, then the back, then move from the wrist up to the elbow, again always moving upwards. Continue along the upper arm, from the elbow towards the shoulder. Repeat on the left side, starting with the hand.

Very gently, brush the abdomen in a clockwise circle. Repeat several times but with a gentler pressure; stop if it feels uncomfortable in any way. Continue on to the chest and neck, always working towards your heart and with gentle pressure.

ALTERNATING SHOWERS

These hydrotherapy showers are a guaranteed way to wake you up! Because the water alternates between hot and cold, the effect is to stimulate the circulation of the blood and lymph, as well as the nervous system and immune system, so that you are less vulnerable to every passing infection.

It takes a little courage the first time that you stand under the cold water so, to start with, have only as much time under the cold shower as you can bear and do it just once. After the first few sessions you will find that the cold water is pleasantly invigorating. At this point you can start building up to longer periods under the cold water and repeat the hot and cold routine up to three times.

Your energy levels will benefit all day long from this treatment. Some naturopaths and beauty experts believe that hydrotherapy showers are powerfully anti-ageing – another good reason to incorporate them into your life.

HOW TO USE ALTERNATING SHOWERS

Start with skin-brushing (see pp. 82–3) or a salt body scrub (pp. 84–5), as this will encourage the elimination of toxins and will improve the texture of the skin. If you want to wash with soap or shower gel or to wash your hair, do this in the first hot session so that you spend most of the time under pure water.

When you have finished skin-brushing or your salt body scrub, turn on the shower so that the water is warm to hot. Get under the shower and let the water pour over you for 2–3 minutes, making sure that your whole body (including your face and head) is covered by the water.

Turn the tap to cool or, if you can stand it, cold (build up to this gradually) and let it cover your whole body for

15–30 seconds, or up to a minute when you are used to it. Turn the water back to hot for another 2–3 minutes, then back to cold. Alternate up to three times and always finish with cold water. It is very beneficial for the complexion to turn your head so that the cold water pours on to your face (see Affusions on pp. 136–7).

Get out and wrap yourself in warm towels. Pat yourself dry and put on a warm dressing gown, then sit or lie down for at least 5 minutes, and ideally up to half an hour.

COLD SHOWERS

Cold showers are often regarded as punitive. However, just as with the cold part of alternating showers, the body quickly accustoms itself to them. There is increasing medical evidence that, taken on a regular basis, just as Vincent Priessnitz believed, these have a strengthening effect on the whole system and build up immunity to infection in a few months. To achieve this, you need to take a daily cold shower lasting only a minute or two. However, in the long term, alternating showers will have much the same effect.

WATER QUALITY

One potential problem with either alternating or hot showers is that many of the less desirable chemicals to be found in tap water can be inhaled as they vaporize in hot water. This is one of the most potent arguments for filtering the water supply to your home (see pp. 28–9).

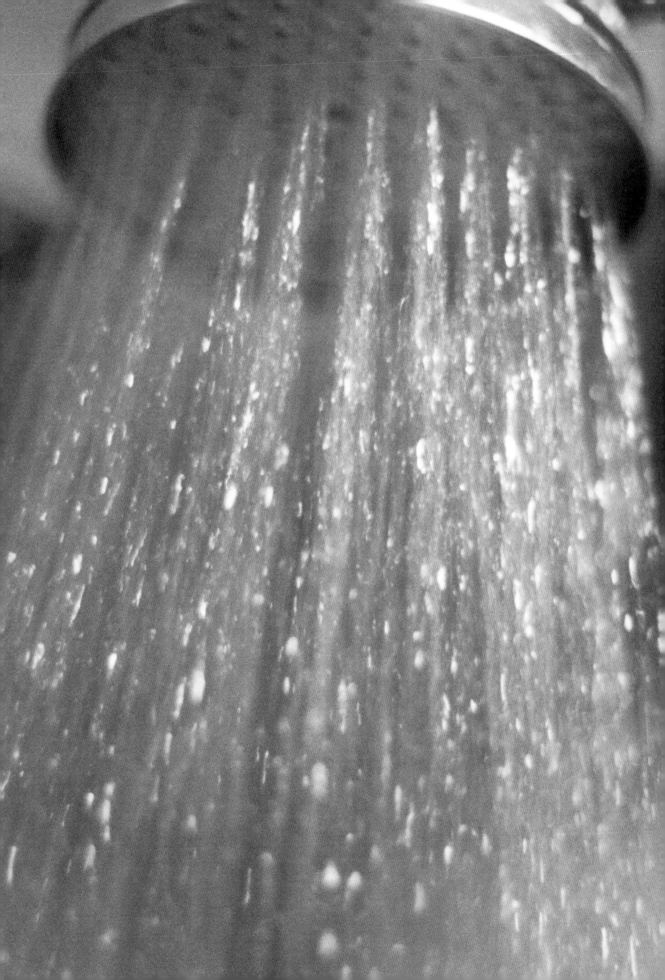

THERAPEUTIC BATHS

There are a number of spa baths that work equally well in the home and are very easy to set up. The extra ingredients that these baths use (if any) are cheap and easily available and yet the results can be extremely beneficial.

HOT AND WARM BATHS

Ordinary baths of various temperatures can be highly effective for particular conditions. A hot bath, for instance – because it encourages blood flow to the part of the body that is submerged – can be soothing for period pains, lower back pain, constipation or haemorrhoids. You should keep the bath shallow, so that only the area you want targeted is in the water. Alternatively, use a sitz bath (see pp. 96–7). Warm baths are very good for the release of tension in the body and work well if you have a problem sleeping. In this case, you would use a full bath of tepid water, staying in it for up to 30 minutes, just before you go to bed.

COLD BATHS

Cold baths are not suitable for the very young, the old or the frail. Even undertaken by the hardiest individual,

this is a treatment to which you should accustom yourself slowly. The underlying principle is the same as that for cold showers – taken over an extended period, there is a gradual build-up of the strength of the immune system and an improvement in the circulation. Even though the water that you use is cold, the bathroom itself should be warm, with plenty of soft towels to hand.

Exposure to cold water should build up very gradually and the whole process may take weeks or even months. Begin by standing in cold water up to your ankles and walking in the water for a few minutes. After a few weeks you can try sitting in the water. Then, after several more weeks, try lying in it up to your neck. The arms and legs should be moving constantly during these stages. In all cases, as soon as you are dry do some simple exercises (such as running on the spot) to warm the body up quickly. Alternatively, try a cold sitz bath (see pp. 96–7).

HEATING BATHS

One of the best baths for general detoxification uses Epsom salts. This may sound like a very old-fashioned treatment, but it is one of the most cleansing and relaxing you can have. The magnesium in the Epsom salts warms and soothes the body, which helps the joints and muscles unwind. It is more than just warming, though. In fact, you can expect to get very hot indeed and, as your temperature rises, you will sweat out your toxic overload.

WATER WISDOM

Too much salt in the diet leads to an imbalance of potassium and to water retention, bloating and, it is believed, in many cases to high blood pressure and cardiovascular disease.

HOW TO USE A HEATING BATH

Epsom salts are available at pharmacies and health-food shops. They usually come in 4lb or 2kg packs.

Throw the whole pack of Epsom salts into the bath. It takes quite a lot of stirring to mix them all in, but it is important that they have dissolved before you get in. If you have difficulty tracking Epsom salts down, you can substitute a handful of herbs or a spoonful of spices – ginger, sage and cayenne pepper have a similar effect in terms of raising the temperature!

Whatever you are using as your heating agent, lie in the bath for at least 15 minutes. You can expect to sweat copiously, but this is just part of the detoxifying process.

You can increase the heating effect by massaging your body with a loofah or bath mitt. As always, start with your feet and use circular movements. Work your way up your legs, buttocks and gently over the abdomen. Massage the upper torso – but not the breasts – and as much as you can of your back.

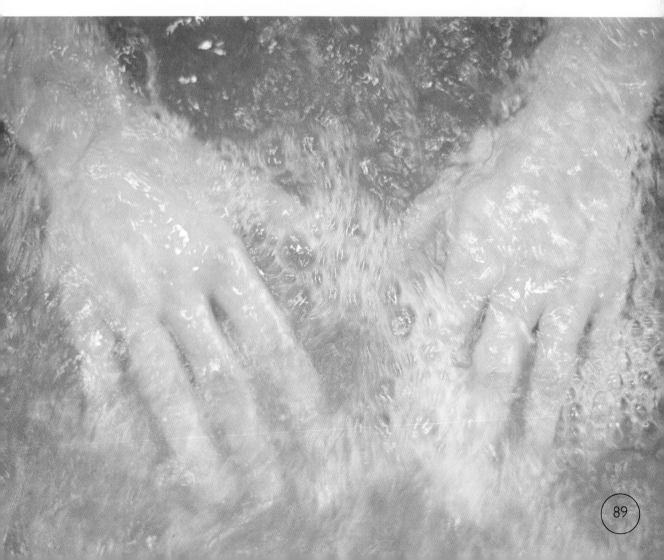

MOOR MUD

Mud may not be one of the most glamorous forms of treatment in the world, but it is one of the oldest. Mud packs were used by the ancient Egyptians and Romans for various ailments and as beauty treatments, and similar treatments have always been available at hydrotherapy spas, most notably in Europe. Therapeutic mud often comes from the areas around mineral springs, and its high mineral content is advanced as one of the main reasons for its remarkable properties – there is growing medical evidence to support this.

NEYDHARTING MOOR MUD

One of the most famous sources of therapeutic mud is the Neydharting Moor, about 37 miles/60km from Salzburg in Austria. Archaeological finds there have shown that the mud was in use from as early as 800 BC by the Celts, followed by the Romans. Sick and injured animals were – and still are – drawn there by its healing powers. The German physician Paracelsus (1493–1541) thought that in this mud he had discovered the 'elixir of life'. There is a thriving clinic at Neydharting today, which is so renowned throughout Europe that there is a long waiting list and its treatments are available on health insurance.

Known just as 'Moor' or 'Moor-Life', the Neydharting mud has been analysed by over 500 scientists and declared to be unique. Because the 20,000-year-old glacial valley basin in which the moor lies was formerly a lake, from which the waters have never fully been drained, the mud has retained all of its invaluable organic, mineral and trace elements. It is especially rich in decomposed plant life and, of its over 1,000 plant deposits – flowering herbs, seeds, leaves, flowers, tubers, fruits, roots and grasses – some 300 have recognized medical properties. Many of these plants are now

extinct; others are not known to exist, or to have ever existed, anywhere else in the world.

According to Moor users, the mud works in a threefold process. First, it detoxifies; then it heals; finally it strengthens the whole system. Medical evidence shows that its properties are both anti-inflammatory and astringent, making it particularly useful for detoxification, for treating skin disorders such as acne, eczema and psoriasis, and for rheumatism and arthritis. Moor has also been used for hormonal and infertility problems and for healing open wounds.

Moor therapists practise in the United States and throughout Europe, as well as at the clinic in Austria, and you can also buy Moor products to use at home. These include oil, mud packs and beauty treatments, such as a cleansing bar and body lotion. The two most widely used products are the Moor bath and the Moor drink. Drinking mud admittedly does not sound very appetizing – and the drink actually does look like mud! It also initially has a strong smell, so it is best left to breathe overnight in a cool room. However, it has neither taste nor odour after that, so a teaspoonful can be mixed into a glass of water or with some fruit.

HOW TO USE A MOOR BATH

The Moor bath treatment comes in a large can that resembles a motor-oil container; again, it does look exactly like real mud.

Mix the Moor bath product well with the water of your bath, or it will form little globules on the surface and will not be nearly so effective.

Your bath water should be warm, not hot. Stay in it for at least half an hour, topping it up with warm water as necessary. This is not a bath to wash in, so do not use any soaps or shampoos. If necessary, take a shower first, then let yourself soak in the mud bath.

Moor has a beneficial effect on all skin, so you can quite happily get your face wet with Moor water – and the same goes for your hair.

Afterwards, pat yourself dry, then rest for at least half an hour. Or, best of all, have a Moor bath late at night, then go to bed straight away – it is a highly relaxing bath and you will usually sleep particularly well after it.

AROMATHERAPY BATHS

One of the most sensually appealing of water treatments is bathing with aromatherapy oils. Not only are you immersed in warm water, but the oil has beneficial effects on your skin and you are surrounded with the loveliest scents. You can choose between any number of oils and effects: bright, enlivening citrus to wake you up; sweet, floral essences to soothe tensions; or exotic, spicy, aphrodisiac scents.

One of the most popular uses of aromatherapy oils is as a relaxant. A number of oils are effective in relaxing body and mind, especially when used in the bath. Last thing at night, an aromatherapy bath can help relax tense muscles, soothe headaches and anxieties, and prepare you for a restful sleep. Even if you do not suffer from insomnia, most people at some point in their lives have a temporary problem with light, restless sleep, which leaves them feeling tired and irritable. This can lead to tension headaches or general aches and pains. NOTE: *Some aromatherapy oils should not be used if you are pregnant. Consult your doctor first.*

HOW TO CREATE AN AROMATHERAPY BATH

An aromatherapy bath is a good way of slowing down the mind and relaxing the body at the end of the day. For the best results, make it a real pleasure.

Prepare the room in advance to make the occasion as tranquil as possible. The bathroom should be warm, as should the towels – make sure they are close at hand for when you get out. Lighting is important, too. Make it as low as possible – candlelight has a wonderfully calming effect and candles scented with relaxing oils are widely available, so you could try one of these.

Fill the bath with water (it should not be too hot or the oil will simply evaporate) and, when it is ready, add 5–10 drops of your chosen oil to the water and stir it around so that it is well mixed in.

Stay in the bath for at least 20 minutes and relax. If it helps you to unwind you can listen to music – make sure it is something soft and tranquil.

When you get out of the bath, wrap yourself in a big, warm towel, but do not dry yourself vigorously. Pat yourself gently with the towel or sit wrapped up in it until it absorbs the water on your body. In this way you keep a little of the oil on your skin.

Put on a dressing gown or pyjamas, then get into bed straight away in order to stay warm and relaxed.

RELAXING OILS

For a relaxing bath that will promote a deep, restful sleep, choose one of the following oils:

Lavender   One of the gentlest oils, so safe that you can apply it directly to the skin, even that of young children. It is a soporific and relieves headaches and both physical and mental stress. If you have trouble sleeping, you can put a drop or two of lavender oil on your pillow or very gently apply it to your temples.

Neroli   Extracted from the blossom of the orange tree, this has a quite sensational smell. It lifts the spirits, as well as being generally calming and is particularly beneficial for mature skin.

Sandalwood   Has a warm, woody fragrance and is an anti-depressant, as well as a soporific. Men often find this more appealing than floral scents and it is used in many men's toiletries.

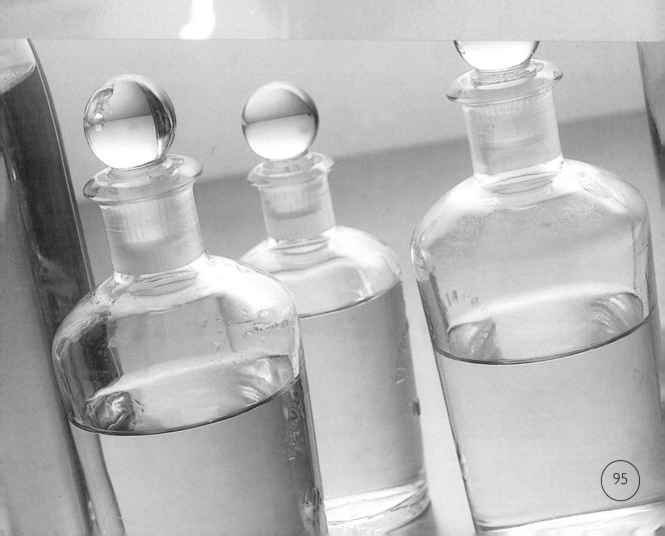

FOOT TREATMENTS, SITZ BATHS AND INHALATIONS

Foot baths of warm or hot water are a simple but effective way of soothing tired feet and ankles. With an added drop of lavender or rose oil, they are particularly pleasant and relaxing. Foot baths can be used for other problems, too.

A mustard bath is an old-fashioned but effective way of stopping a headache before it has really taken hold. Simply add a teaspoonful of mustard powder to a washing-up bowl of hot water and put your feet in it, at the same time putting a cold compress on your forehead. Relax as much as you can and keep your feet in the bath for 20–30 minutes. And immersing just the hands and feet in cold water for 5 minutes immediately before going to bed is thought to be beneficial for insomnia.

SITZ BATHS

You can set up your own version of a sitz bath in much the same way. These are particularly useful for abdominal or gynaecological problems, as well as being a general tonic. You will need to use two bowls (large washing-up bowls or baby baths, for instance) and put very cold water in one and water as hot as you can bear in the other (though obviously not scalding). Then put your feet in the cold water and sit in the hot water; alternate the two and finish by sitting in the cold. A cold sitz bath last thing at night is recommended for insomnia. Your upper body should be warmly dressed and you just sit in the water for a matter of seconds – a minute at most. Dry yourself quickly afterwards and get straight into bed. Even more unexpectedly, a cold sitz bath is recommended for relieving congestion due to hay fever.

INHALATIONS

Inhalations are well known as a means of removing congestion and the worst symptoms of colds and sinus problems. They are, of course, very simple to set up at home, as all you need is a bowl, a towel and a kettle. If you are using this treatment for congestion, a drop or two of eucalyptus oil mixed in with the water is remarkably effective.

Simply fill the bowl with boiling water, add the oil and lean over the bowl. Cover your head with the towel so that it forms a tent over the bowl and inhale deeply for several minutes. This treatment is not, however, suitable for asthmatics.

WATER WISDOM

Britain suffers from over-abstraction of water. So in the last 20 years we have had 3 droughts, when only one would normally be expected every 200 years.

HOW TO WATER-TREAD

Water-treading is a very well-known hydrotherapy spa treatment and at some spas you go outside to walk through an icy running stream. At home, however, you can set this up in the bathroom.

Fill the bath with very cold water – you can even throw some ice cubes in, if you like – so that it is at the right level to reach over your ankles. Once you are used to it, it can come up to your calves.

With the rest of your body fully and warmly clothed, bare your legs from the knee down and stand in the bath.

Walk on the spot so that the feet alternately come right out of the water with each step. Try to feel as if you are going right through the foot – toes, instep, heel – each time. To start with, you should stay in the water for only 30 seconds, but over time you can build up to 2 or 3 minutes.

When you have finished, get out and dry the feet and ankles, then put on thick (preferably warmed-up) socks. Rest for 10 minutes or so. Alternatively, do this at bedtime and go to bed immediately afterwards – water-treading is excellent for light, interrupted sleep and for insomnia generally.

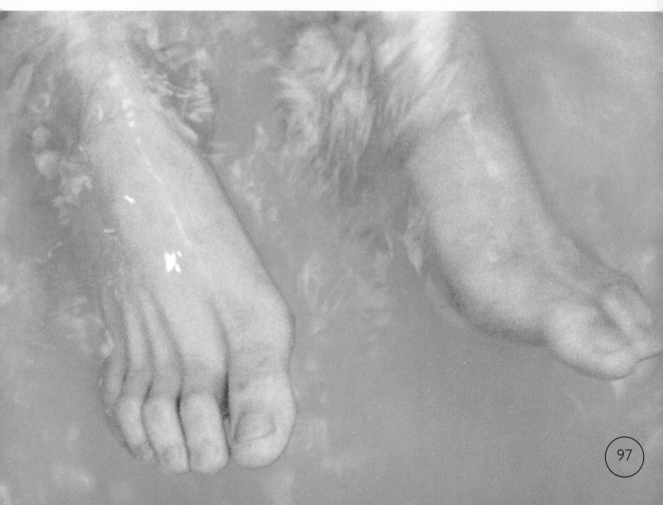

AILMENT DIRECTORY

There is a very wide variety of ailments that can be treated using hydrotherapy. This chart shows self-help treatments and those that can be carried out easily at home. However, if you have a serious ailment, or are in any doubt about what it is or about your state of health generally, always consult your medical practitioner. Increased water intake is beneficial to just about all of these ailments, incidentally.

STRESS AND ANXIETY	A wide range of hydrotherapy treatments is suitable, including swimming and water therapy exercises, heat treatments such as saunas and steam baths, flotation tanks and water massage.
FATIGUE AND INSOMNIA	These tend to go hand-in-hand, for obvious reasons. Try alternating showers in the morning and alternating sitz baths at night. Warm baths are also beneficial, especially with the addition of Moor mud or essential oils, such as lavender or rose.
LOW SEX DRIVE, FERTILITY PROBLEMS, IMPOTENCE	Cold sitz baths at night. Really!
HEADACHES AND MIGRAINE	Hot mustard baths for the feet and cold compresses for the forehead, to which a drop of lavender oil may be added.
COLDS AND FLU	Steam inhalation with eucalyptus oil for congestion. If you can catch a cold before it really takes hold, a sauna can sometimes stop it in its tracks. Alternating showers will build up your immunity.
ASTHMA	Regular swimming, but not breaststroke.
RHEUMATISM, ARTHRITIS, JOINT PROBLEMS	Water exercises, if done regularly, will help free up joints. Use a hot pack – a towel soaked in hot water, then wrung out– applied directly to badly inflamed joints to bring down the swelling. Dead Sea and Moor baths and flotation tanks may also be beneficial.

BACKACHE	Flotation tanks, water massage or hydrotherapy baths.
CRAMP, POOR CIRCULATION	Skin-brushing, salt body scrubs, alternating showers.
HIGH BLOOD PRESSURE	Flotation tanks, alternating showers.
MENSTRUAL PROBLEMS, URINARY INFECTIONS	Alternating sitz baths. Try an aromatherapy bath with two drops each of lavender, juniper berry, eucalyptus and sandalwood oils for cystitis.
CONSTIPATION	Hot sitz baths.
FLUID RETENTION	Moor bath, Dead Sea bath, Epsom salts bath or aromatherapy bath with two drops each of juniper berry and eucalyptus oils.
CELLULITE	Skin-brushing, alternating showers, steam baths, Epsom salts bath.
ACNE	Steam baths, facial steamer, affusions.
ECZEMA AND PSORIASIS	Moor bath, Dead Sea bath, Epsom salts bath, steam baths, alternating showers.
LOCALIZED PAIN (including toothache, earache or a sprain)	Ice pack.
VARICOSE VEINS, HAEMORRHOIDS	Alternating sitz baths.

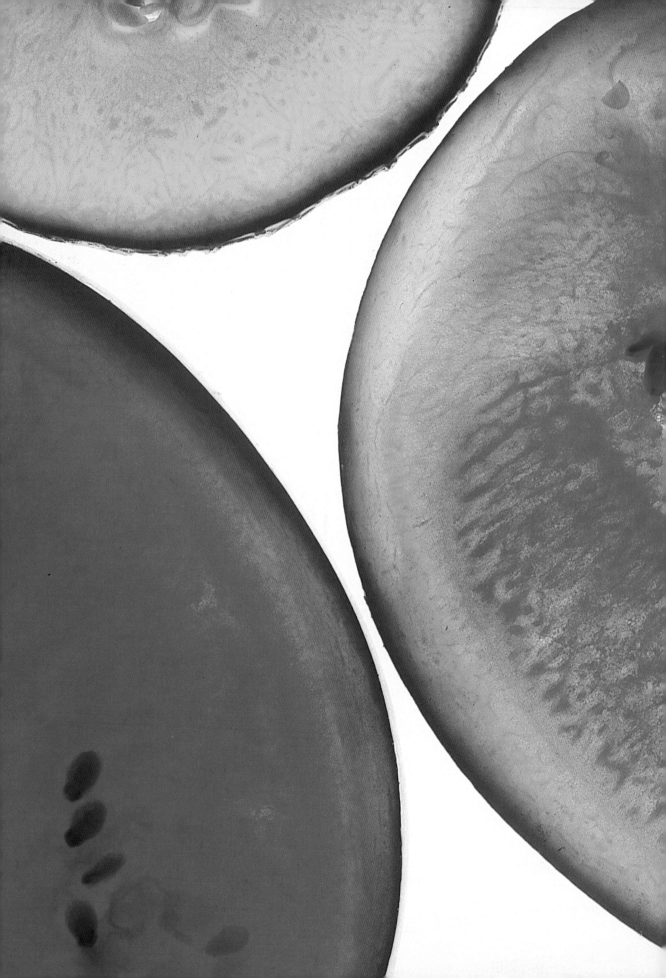

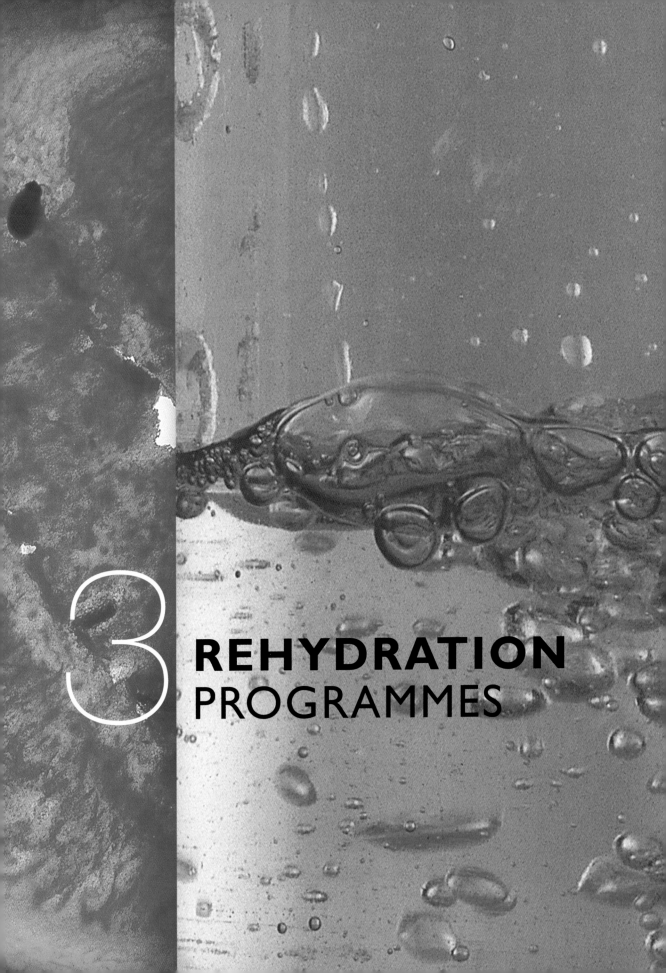

3 REHYDRATION PROGRAMMES

THE **PROGRAMMES**

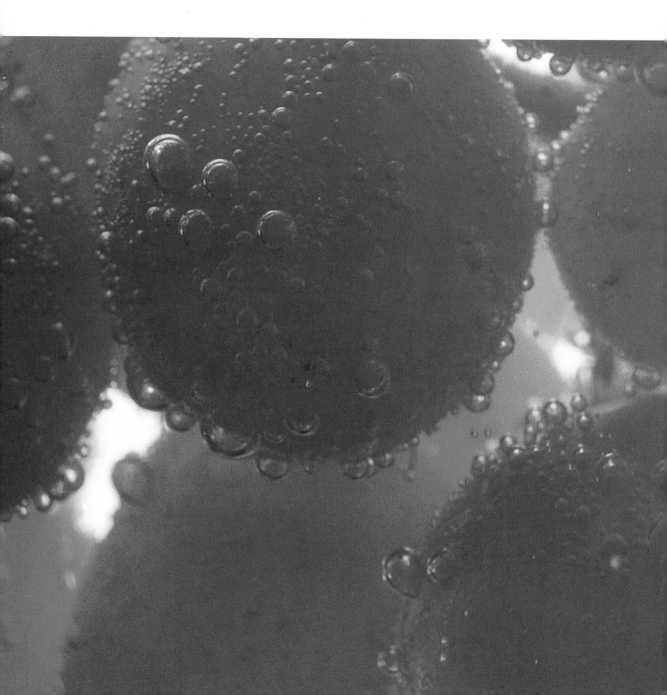

The two programmes in this section of the book offer two different approaches to rehydration. The Weekend Programme begins on a Friday evening and lasts until Sunday evening. The One-Month Programme lasts an entire 4 weeks. While both will increase your internal water level, the Weekend Programme is designed to rid your body generally of toxins, with a deeply cleansing diet and treatments. The One-Month Programme aims to raise hydration levels on a permanent basis in every area of your life, including your environment.

You can repeat the Weekend Programme whenever you have the time or the inclination. It works as a good detox whenever you feel as if you have been overdoing it and is highly relaxing. For the One-Month Programme you obviously need to make a greater commitment in terms of time. However, except for the first week when you do need to concentrate on diet, it is a very gradual plan and is quite easy to absorb into your normal life.

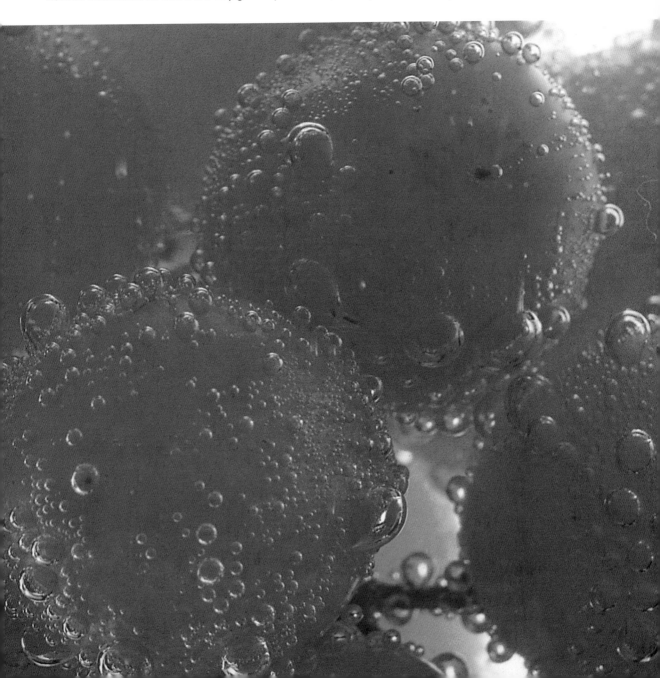

THE WEEKEND PROGRAMME

This is a programme that both detoxifies and rehydrates, and it makes an excellent all-round pick-me-up sometimes when you feel you've been overindulging or if you're feeling tired and stressed. To get the most out of it, choose a weekend when you can devote yourself to it, either on your own or with a friend who will do the programme with you. Do not try to fit it around your normal weekend routine – it simply will not work.

The diet for the weekend course is deeply cleansing, so your body will be throwing off toxins rapidly. Make sure that you drink at least as much water as the programme suggests, so that these toxins will be lost quickly and with as few side-effects as possible.

During any detoxification process, as the body rids itself of long-stored poisons you will inevitably feel the effects. The theory is that the toxins we take into our bodies have a double sting – once on the way in and once on the way out. These can vary from headaches to skin eruptions and digestive upsets. However, because of the gentle treatments used on this programme and the large amount of water that you consume, such side-effects are kept to a minimum. With luck you will not feel any ill-effects at all, but if you do get a headache try

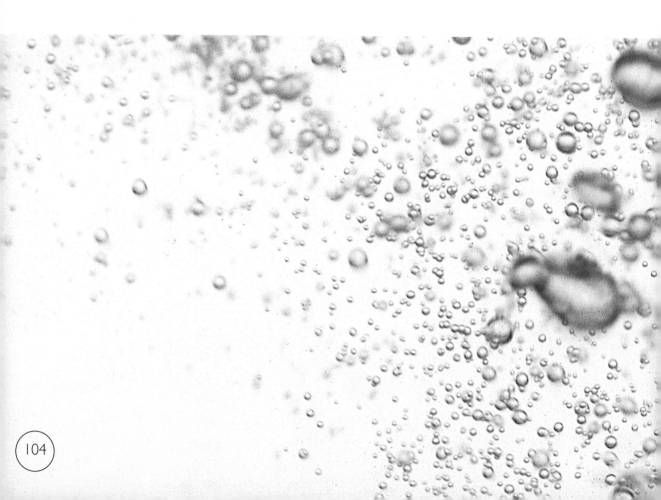

to avoid taking painkillers. Drink lots more water, then lie down and rest, using a lavender compress (see p. 112), if you wish.

Rest is, in fact, another extremely important element of the weekend and will help in the detox process. If you get enough rest, your body can concentrate on its deep cleansing work and you will feel much more relaxed and refreshed. So try to get to bed at the suggested time, even if it seems much earlier than usual.

There is exercise to do, too, and the weekend has a very particular pattern, designed to slow you down and relax you on Friday and Saturday and then, on Sunday, begin to energize you for the week to come.

There are some 'don'ts' on this weekend – things you really must avoid if the programme is going to work. All of the drinks discussed in Chapter One – tea, coffee, fizzy drinks, alcohol (see pp. 20–22) – are off-limits, because they will counteract the rehydration process and give the liver new toxins to process just when it needs to concentrate on getting rid of what is already stored in the body.

Cigarettes are banned, for obvious reasons, and if you do currently smoke, this weekend can in itself be quite a good way to encourage yourself to stop. Food quality should be high – stick to the recommended diet and, if you can, buy organic food.

Above all, listen to what your body has to tell you. If you feel tired, rest, even if it is the middle of the day. Go at your own pace and take your time over the treatments. One of the great benefits in a busy world is that this is a weekend that is all about *you*. Enjoy it.

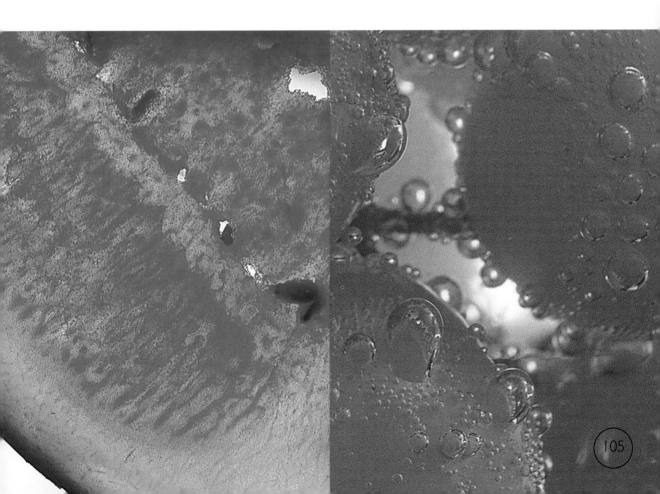

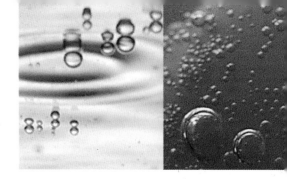

FRIDAY NIGHT

This weekend is for you – so give yourself the chance to reap the maximum benefit from it. Do not make any commitments to other people. If you have young children, ask a friend or grandparent to take them for a sleepover. If you have been working all week, try to switch off completely from the office and its stresses. The more you can rest and relax, the better the programme will work.

Prepare in advance for the weekend by buying everything you will need the preceding week. Check through the recipes for the whole weekend (including teas, herbs and water quantities) and make sure that you have all you will need. There are various extras you require – oils, rock salt, body brush, bath products, and so on – but again, shop for these in advance.

The earlier you can start on Friday, the better. Realistically, however, it will probably be six or seven o'clock in the evening before you are able to focus on yourself. To prepare for the weekend, try to drink extra water during the day on Friday. The first thing to do when you are actually ready to start the programme is to drink a whole glass of water. (All the glasses of water referred to during the weekend are 8fl oz/250ml in size and they should always be filtered or spring water.)

The weekend's food is all light, easily digested and detoxifying. Even so, the earlier you eat, the better. If

FRIDAY EVENING SCHEDULE

The evening programme looks something like this, although you may of course have to adjust it according to your own starting time:

6 p.m.	Drink 8fl oz/250ml water
7 p.m.	Supper
8 p.m.	Drink another 8fl oz/250ml water
9 p.m.	Epsom salts bath (see pp. 88–9)
10 p.m.	Bedtime (have a cup of herbal tea, if you like a hot drink at night)

you eat late, your body will be trying to digest food when you are asleep, when your metabolism should be concentrating instead on the rehydration and detoxification processes. Leave at least an hour – and preferably longer – after eating and before your bath, for the same reason. Relax in the bath, pat yourself dry, then hop into bed for an early night – the bath virtually guarantees a deep, restful sleep.

SUPPER

Tonight's supper should be light and nutritious and, like all this weekend's recipes, low in salt, since salt puts a great strain on your already overworked kidneys. Here are two suggestions – one hot, one cold. Also bear in mind that you need to start preparing tomorrow morning's muesli tonight (see pp. 108–9), as you will on the next two evenings.

CARROT SOUP

This is delicious and very warming, so it makes a good recipe for a chilly winter's night. Serve with wholemeal bread. This recipe makes enough for two servings, although if you are feeling really hungry you may want a second helping. Alternatively, freeze the remainder for another evening.

9oz/250g carrots

1 potato

17fl oz/500ml water or vegetable stock

1 garlic clove, chopped

1oz/25g fresh parsley, chopped

1/2 teaspoon each of fresh sage and thyme, chopped

1/2 teaspoon vegetable extract

pinch of cayenne pepper

Scrub and roughly chop the carrots and potato, then place in a large saucepan with the water or stock and bring to the boil. Add the chopped garlic and all the herbs, the vegetable extract and cayenne and simmer for 20 minutes. Blend in a food processor until smooth, reheat and serve.

SUPER-SALAD

Again, this recipe serves two – or one very hungry person – and it is packed with powerful vitamins and minerals. Do not store salad, for it goes sad, so just make as much as you will need. Serve with wholemeal bread.

2oz/50g rocket

2oz/50g watercress

2oz/50g lamb's lettuce or dandelion leaves

1/2 red onion, sliced

1 small avocado, peeled, stoned and sliced

1oz/25g toasted sesame and sunflower seeds

FOR THE DRESSING

1 tablespoon olive oil

1 teaspoon wholegrain mustard

1 teaspoon lemon juice

salt (a pinch or none at all) and black pepper

Wash and roughly tear up all the leaves and place in a large bowl. Add the onion, avocado and seeds. Mix together. Put all the dressing ingredients in a jar and shake to combine, then pour over the salad.

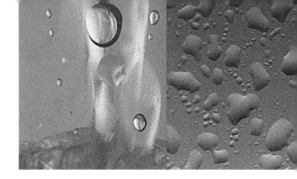

SATURDAY MORNING

After your Epsom Salts bath and an early night you should wake up feeling very refreshed. This morning begins with gentle exercise to stimulate the lymphatic system, followed by a salt body scrub to encourage further elimination through the skin; increased water levels to help rehydration; and a light lunch.

SATURDAY MORNING SCHEDULE

Depending on what time you wake up, the schedule looks something like this:

8 a.m.	Drink 8fl oz/250ml water as soon as you wake up; this will help as a detoxification aid for your kidneys and liver
8.30 a.m.	It is always preferable to exercise before you eat, so do a few gentle yoga stretches (see below); have another glass of water when you finish
9 a.m.	Do your salt body scrub now (see pp. 84–5), finishing with a cool shower for 30–60 seconds; pat yourself dry and wrap up in a warm dressing gown
9.30 a.m.	Drink another glass of water now
10 a.m.	Breakfast, then relax for at least an hour
11 a.m.	Herbal tea
11.30 a.m.	Drink another glass of water now – more if you wish
12.00	Lunch

YOGA STRETCHES

Triangle

1. Stand with your feet about 3ft/90cm apart, your back straight and your shoulders down. Breathe in and lift your arms to shoulder height, turning your feet so that the right foot points out to the side, with the left straight ahead.

2. As you breathe out, bend at the waist and take your right hand down your right leg as far as you can towards the foot, without straining.

3. Raise your left arm so that your fingers are pointing to the ceiling, palm facing forwards. Turn your face to look up into the hand and breathe normally. Hold for as long as possible (up to 3 minutes), then repeat on the other side.

Cobra

1. Lie face down on the floor with your legs together and your hands flat on the floor, so that the tips of your fingers are in line with your shoulders. As you inhale, raise your head, then your shoulders and chest as far as you can from the floor, with your arms bearing the weight.

2. Breathe out and try to stretch further. Breathe normally for several breaths, then lower yourself to the ground.

Shoulder-stand

1. Lie flat on the floor on your back, legs together and arms at your sides. Breathe in and bend your knees to your chest.

2. As you breathe out, raise your lower back from the floor, supporting your hips with your hands. Roll up until your feet are pointing to the ceiling, making your back and legs one long, straight line. Hold and breathe naturally, trying to relax into the position.

3. If you wish, you can now take this shoulder-stand into the plough position by gently lowering your feet behind your head as far as you can – ideally with the toes resting on the ground. Again, try to relax into the position. From either position return to lying flat on the floor.

4. Relax for at least 5 minutes.

BREAKFAST: BIRCHER-BENNER MUESLI

This is nothing like the muesli you buy in supermarkets, which tends to be heavily grain-based. Instead, this muesli is fruit-based. It was invented by the renowned Swiss physician and naturopath, Max Bircher-Benner, in the early twentieth century.

2 tablespoons porridge oats

2 tablespoons sultanas

4 tablespoons fruit juice (apple or pineapple)

1 apple or pear

1 banana

1 tablespoon chopped mixed nuts

$^1/_2$ teaspoon ground ginger

TO SERVE

2 tablespoons live yoghurt

1 teaspoon honey

On Friday night, soak the oats and sultanas in the fruit juice. The following morning grate the apple or pear, slice the banana and mix them into the oats with the nuts and ginger. To serve, add honey if you wish and top with yoghurt.

LUNCH

For lunch, choose either the soup or salad recipe from Friday evening (see pp. 106–7) or one of the Saturday-evening recipes (see pp. 112–13).

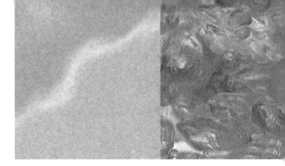

SATURDAY EVENING

By now you should be feeling much more relaxed and cleansed than you did this time yesterday. The detoxifying and rehydrating processes are well under way and will be further accelerated by tonight's bath. Try to get to bed early again, preferably straight after your bath, as this will concentrate the body's energies on its important tasks.

If you do get a headache, try not to take any drugs for pain relief. Instead, use a lavender compress: soak a clean piece of cotton fabric in ice-cold water to which 4 drops of lavender essential oil have been added. Leave it to soak for a few minutes, then wring it out and place it across the forehead. Lie down and relax. Other good oils for a headache are rose and peppermint.

Supper is early again. Choose from the recipes given below, or repeat those from yesterday. If you wish, you can make double the quantity of lentil and celery soup and save some for Sunday; or make something new each time. If you would like to finish with something sweet, have some more fruit. Don't forget to prepare your muesli for tomorrow morning.

SATURDAY EVENING SCHEDULE

5.30 p.m.	Have a glass of water while you prepare supper
6 p.m.	Supper
7 p.m.	Drink another glass of water before your bath; if drinking very close to bedtime means that you wake up in the night to go to the lavatory, make this your last drink of the day
8 p.m.	Take a Moor mud, seaweed or Dead Sea salts bath (see pp. 90–93); stay in for a minimum of half an hour, but preferably an hour, topping up with hot water as necessary. Do not use soap or any other sort of cleanser in this bath. If you want to shampoo your hair, do that first in the shower. When you get out of the bath, pat yourself dry so that you do not remove all of the minerals, which will continue to be absorbed by your skin throughout the night.
9.30 p.m.	Have a last glass of water or a herbal tea (optional)
10 p.m.	Bedtime

PASTA WITH CHILLI TOMATO SAUCE

The chillies make this a warming dish, but you can cool it down by adding more yoghurt. The sauce will make enough for three to four servings, but it can be kept in the fridge for later use. Add a green salad, if you wish.

1 onion

1 red chilli

1 garlic clove

2 tablespoons olive oil

1 large tin tomatoes in their own juice

2 tablespoons tomato purée

salt (just a pinch) and black pepper

TO SERVE (ONE PORTION)

3oz/75g wholemeal pasta

2–4 tablespoons live yoghurt

Chop the onion and chilli and crush the garlic, then fry gently in the olive oil. When the onion is soft, add the tomatoes and the purée, together with the salt and pepper. Meanwhile, cook the pasta in boiling, lightly salted water until *al dente*, then drain. Arrange the pasta on a plate, pour over the sauce and spoon over the yoghurt.

LENTIL AND CELERY SOUP

This recipe makes four servings, so you can keep some for tomorrow or freeze the rest and use it at a later date. Serve with wholemeal bread.

1 onion

3 celery sticks

1 garlic clove

2 tablespoons olive oil

6oz/175g red lentils

2pints/1.2 litres vegetable stock

1/2 teaspoon cayenne pepper

salt (a pinch only) and black pepper

TO SERVE (ONE PORTION)

1 tablespoon live natural yoghurt

Chop the onion and celery and crush the garlic. Heat the oil in a saucepan and add the vegetables, simmering gently until the onion softens. Add the lentils and the stock, bring to the boil and simmer for 20 minutes. Check the seasoning, adding cayenne, salt and pepper as necessary. Spoon over the yoghurt to serve.

SUNDAY MORNING

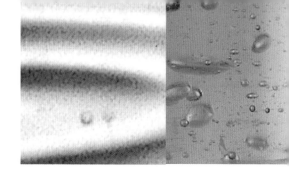

Start the day with a large cup of hot water. You can have it plain or, if you like, you can add a squeeze of lemon for flavour; if you prefer sweetness, add a teaspoonful of organic honey. Go back to bed with this or sit quietly – try to start the day gently. Before your hydrotherapy showers and skin-brushing, wake up your mind and body for the day by repeating Saturday morning's exercises – with a few extras today, if you wish (see below). After you have exercised, drink another cup of hot water, or a glass of cold if you prefer.

At some point during the day you may want to visit your local pool or health club – this would be particularly good if they have steam rooms or saunas. You could go this morning and combine an exercise class (nothing too vigorous, though) or a swim with a steam or sauna, instead of the exercises and hydrotherapy showers at home. If you do this, take your brush with you and do some skin-brushing before you have your steam or sauna.

If you go in the afternoon, just have a swim and, if it is available, a massage – particularly a lymphatic drainage one – or a mud or seaweed treatment. If you do not feel up to doing any of these, try going for a walk after breakfast, somewhere pleasant: in the countryside, in a park or, best of all, by the sea. If you feel very tired, simply follow the schedule below and rest as much as you can, as that will clearly be of most benefit to you.

SUNDAY MORNING SCHEDULE

7 a.m.	Drink a large cup of hot water with lemon and/or honey (see above); rest for a little while, as you drink
7.30 a.m.	Yoga stretches (see pages 108–9 and below)
8.30 a.m.	Drink another cup of hot or cold water before your skin-brushing and hydrotherapy showers; if you cannot wait for breakfast, have it now, but leave the treatments for at least another hour
9 a.m.	Skin-brushing (see pp. 82–3) and alternating hydrotherapy showers (see pp. 86–7); rest afterwards for at least half an hour and drink another glass of water
10 a.m.	Breakfast, as yesterday
11 a.m.	Glass of water, followed by a walk; rest until lunchtime

YOGA

Begin, as yesterday, with the triangle and the cobra. Then go on to the spine twist, the dog pose, follow with the plough or shoulder-stand and finish with the cat. Lie down and relax for at least 10 minutes when you have finished the exercises.

The spine twist

1. Sit with a straight back and your legs straight out in front of you. Take your left leg over the right and place the left foot next to the right knee.

2. Put your right hand on your left thigh and turn your body towards the left, so that you feel as if you are twisting around your spine. Place your left hand behind you for balance and hold the twist for at least a minute, breathing normally. Repeat on the other side.

Dog pose

1. Stand up straight with your feet together. Raise your arms so that your fingertips are pointing at the ceiling.

2. Bend from the waist, keeping your back straight and your arms outstretched, and reaching out in front of you. As you pass waist level, reach towards the floor.

3. Touch the floor with your hands, bending your knees, if necessary. Walk your hands forwards until your arms and legs are stretched out, in a triangle, with your bottom at the apex. Relax the neck and breathe, holding the position for up to a minute.

4. Bend your knees to the floor and roll your back up, so that you sit on your heels before getting up.

The cat

If you have any back problems, miss out the final step.

1. Kneel down with your hands flat on the floor and your arms straight and in line with your hips. Try to make your neck feel as though it extends in one long line from your spine, so that your back looks like a table top.

2. Breathe in and, as you breathe out, pull your navel towards your spine and form a high, open arch with your back, like a cat stretching.

3. Breathe in to return to the table-top position. Then, as you breathe out, drop your back into a concave shape and lift your head to look up to the ceiling. Repeat the whole sequence slowly 4 times. Then relax on the floor.

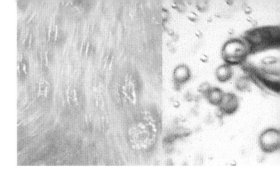

SUNDAY EVENING

By now you should be feeling relaxed, energized and profoundly cleansed. Not only will your increased water intake have affected the functioning of your internal organs and systems, but the results of rehydration should be visible in your skin, too, plumping out fine lines and giving it a new bloom. With benefits like these, you will want to increase your water intake permanently!

The rest of Sunday is highly relaxing, aimed at increasing your well-being and energy levels, so that you start the new week refreshed and raring to go. Try to get an early night again, preferably immediately after your aromatherapy bath, as this will have prepared you for a deep and relaxing sleep.

SUNDAY EVENING SCHEDULE

6 p.m.	Have a glass of water while you prepare supper
6.30 p.m.	Supper
7.30 p.m.	Drink another glass of water before your bath and do not drink another today, if it wakes you during the night
8.30 p.m.	Aromatherapy bath (see below)
9.30 p.m.	Herbal tea or water (optional)
10 p.m.	Bed

AROMATHERAPY BATH

Preparing an aromatherapy bath, and the best oils to use, are explained in full on pp. 94–5. After your bath, pat yourself dry and, if you wish, apply an aromatherapy oil based on the same essence as the one you used in the bath. Put 12 drops of your chosen oil into a glass bottle containing 1fl oz/25ml of carrier oil – grapeseed, almond or peach oils are rich in vitamins and easily absorbed, or you could simply use sunflower or olive oil from the kitchen cupboard. Give the bottle a shake to mix the contents well, then smooth the oil evenly all over your body.

SUPPER

Choose from any of the preceding recipes for the weekend or one of the following. If you would like something sweet afterwards, have some fruit or some natural yoghurt flavoured with honey.

PRAWN RISOTTO

This makes two servings, but it is equally good the next day as a cold salad.

I onion

2 tablespoons olive oil

2oz/125g brown (or basmati) rice

I/₂pt/300ml water

salt (only if you need it – remember that
    prawns are salty) and black pepper

I red pepper, chopped

I garlic clove, chopped

2oz/50g almonds or pine kernels

6oz/175g prawns

Chop the onion finely and fry it in half of the olive oil, until soft. Add the rice and cook for I minute, mixing it with the onion. Then add the water with a pinch of salt and bring to the boil. If you are using brown rice, simmer for around 40 minutes; for basmati rice, 20 minutes. In a frying pan heat the rest of the oil and fry the chopped pepper for 2 minutes. Add the crushed garlic, the almonds or pine kernels and the prawns and fry for 2 more minutes, then stir into the rice and mix together well. Check the seasoning and serve.

LENTIL BURGERS

This recipe will serve two, but you can always freeze the extra for later use. Serve with a salad.

I/₂ onion

olive oil, for frying

6oz/175g red lentils

2oz/50g basmati rice

8fl oz/250ml water

pinch of salt

pinch of turmeric and cumin

pinch of sugar

I tablespoon oatmeal or porridge oats

Chop the onion finely and fry in a little oil. Add the lentils and rice, then the water, salt, spices and sugar. Simmer until the mixture becomes very thick, then leave to cool. Stir in most of the oatmeal or porridge oats, reserving a little for the coating. Sprinkle this on to a plate, form the lentil mixture into patty shapes and roll in the remaining oatmeal or oats. Fry in a little olive oil until browned, then serve immediately.

THE ONE-MONTH PROGRAMME

The One-Month Programme is a gradual programme aimed at rehydrating, cleansing and energizing your life on every level. It deals with your diet (including herbal drinks), your skin, your mind, your exercise regime, your general health and even your home. It may sound like a tall order but it is, in fact, very easy to follow and, once you have started on the right diet and water intake, the benefits begin immediately. After that, other new ideas are introduced each week for you to try.

The first week of the programme is the one that is likely to bring about the most obvious and immediate changes in your life, as it affects your daily diet and water intake. So bear this in mind when you decide to start the programme – choose a week when you will not have too many social or work commitments, which might make it more difficult for you to focus on your health.

The week works as a complete detoxification for all those overworked organs and systems that we looked at in Part One of the book and it starts the programme off with a real boost to your health.

Afterwards you can increase your sense of well-being with exercise, meditation and relaxation, as you establish a routine for maximum health. Specific herbal drinks are

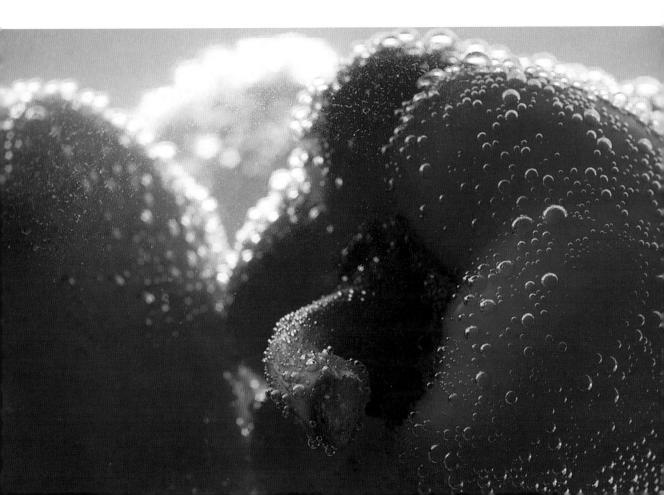

SALT WARNING

All the food you eat on the One-Month Programme should contain either very little added salt or, even better, none at all. Excess salt upsets the regulating of your body fluids and puts strain on the kidneys – just at the time when you are supposed to be giving them a rest. In fact, we all eat far more salt than is good for us (up to ten times as much as we actually need) and a great deal of salt is hidden in processed foods, which is one of the reasons why all of the food on the programme should be freshly prepared. Unfortunately, we all acquire the taste for salt and get into the habit of using it, which means that we take more and more of it all the time. Use this programme to kick the salt habit.

suggested to relieve particular ailments or for particular effects, as well as facial affusions to tighten the skin, which you can use whenever you need them. There is advice on how to incorporate hydrotherapy into your daily life, in order to boost your immune system and ward off infection, and hints on how to make your home a healthier place.

Some of these elements are going to appeal to you more than others; some may not appeal at all. However, if you use just a few of them – including the raised water intake, of course – you will become aware of enormous benefits in the way you feel and the way you look. Increased hydration is perhaps the biggest single boost you can give to your health, and this programme shows you how to achieve it.

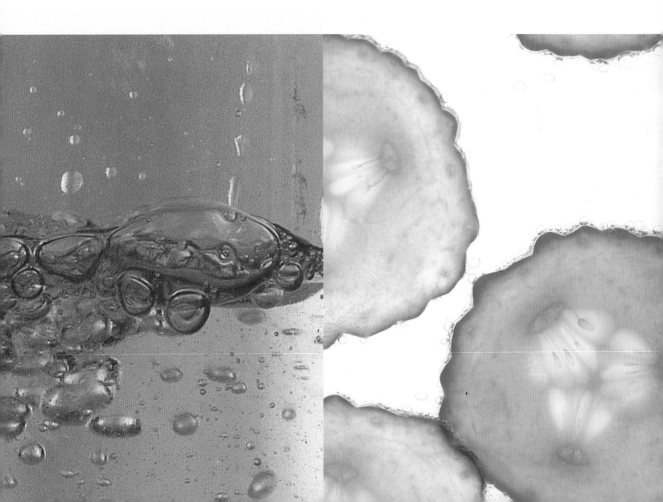

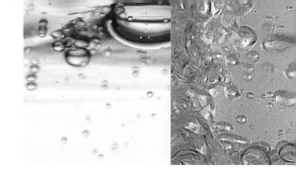

WEEK ONE

The aim of the first week is to relieve the organs of the body that have been suffering from an overload of toxins and to rehydrate them. The way to do this is to increase your intake of water, prevent new toxins entering the body by removing them from your diet, and base the majority of your diet on raw food.

INCREASING WATER INTAKE

This is the most vital aspect of Week One – essential if you are to get the maximum benefit from the programme. The rehydration plan follows exactly the one outlined in the chart on 'Hydration through the day' on pp. 24–5, although you may need to make small changes to it to get it to fit in with your day. However, do make sure that you drink at least 8 glasses of water daily.

DOS AND DON'TS

During this week you need to avoid toxins, as your body is going through a major rehydration and cleansing process, so:

Do avoid tea, coffee and alcohol

Don't smoke cigarettes

Do drink herbal teas (see pp. 130–31) and unsweetened fruit juices, too.

Don't worry about how often this makes you go to the lavatory – it is inevitable! In fact, your body will soon get used to the new rhythm and you will find that your urine is getting paler and thinner – a sure sign that the programme is working.

RAW FOODS

Raw fruit and vegetables are extremely cleansing, particularly for the digestive tract, and also have a high water content to help the rehydration process. So two out of three meals each day should be based on raw food. You can choose which meals will be raw to suit your own routine, but a salad or fruit offers an easy option to take to the office.

The best way to assemble a salad is to go to the market or supermarket and buy those fruits and vegetables that look at their best – ripe, fresh and, whenever possible, organic. You can do this most easily in summer, but even in winter you can make delicious raw salads with varieties of cabbage, root vegetables and beets.

Unless you are tackling a vegetable with a very tough skin (such as swede), scrub it clean with a stiff brush rather than peeling it. Many of the most vital nutrients in vegetables are found just under the skin, so if you peel them, you throw these away. The other way to lose nutrients is through air and water. *Never* leave vegetables to soak in water and always prepare them just before you are ready to eat – the longer they are exposed to the air, the less nutritional value they will actually contain.

Depending on the vegetables that you have bought, you can either toss them together in a salad dressing or arrange them in an attractive pattern on a plate. Keep dressings simple – olive oil, lemon, salt and pepper; or yoghurt with lemon, herbs, salt and pepper – or make a separate dip, such as humus or yoghurt and garlic. In winter (or with root vegetables) add horseradish or mustard to your dressings and dips to spice them up.

Toasted pine nuts, sesame seeds, sunflower seeds or flaked almonds can be thrown on top of the salad and will give it a delicious, distinctive flavour. You can also make a simple rice salad, or have some wholemeal bread with your meal – it does not have to be totally raw and you should certainly not be left feeling hungry.

REHYDRATING VEGETABLES

Year-round raw vegetables

Lettuce (all varieties), radicchio, frisé (curly endive/chicory), watercress, fennel, carrots, cauliflower, broccoli, avocados, radishes, spring onions, onions, garlic, celery, peppers, tomatoes, cucumbers, mushrooms, peas, beets, spinach, chicory, pak-choi, Chinese leaves

---

Winter raw vegetables

Jerusalem artichokes, celeriac, Brussels sprouts, turnips, parsnips, red cabbage, leeks

---

Summer raw vegetables

Lamb's lettuce, cress, dandelion leaves, nasturtium leaves, lovage, vine leaves, beans (runner, string, broad, etc.), mangetout

FRUIT MEALS

Fruit has superb rehydration properties and makes an ideal snack if you want something extra between meals. If you do not think you will feel too hungry, you can have one vegetable salad and one fruit salad as your main meals of the day during Week One. If, however, you think this is going to be too much of a shock to the system, make breakfast your fruit meal and have a cooked main meal either at lunchtime or for dinner.

For breakfast, either have several pieces of fruit – such as melon, watermelon, grapes and apples – or make yourself some Bircher-Benner muesli (see p. 109), which you need to half-prepare the night before. Another alternative, which is especially delicious in winter, is to stew dried fruits (prunes, figs, dried apricots, peaches and dates) in orange juice for about half an hour. Add cloves, cinnamon, nutmeg or ginger, if you like a spicy flavour, but do not forget to remove any cloves before you serve it. You can have some natural yoghurt with any of these options, sweetened with honey if you like.

If you are going to have fruit as one of your main meals, you can either have a large fruit salad – pour a little orange juice over the fruit and add honey, if you wish – served with yoghurt; or separate fruits arranged on a plate.

Cooked meals

During Week One – unless you are used to this sort of diet – it is probably best to have one cooked meal each day. This is especially true if your normal routine is continuing, whether you work in or out of the home. Otherwise, you may find your energy levels dropping too much for you to cope.

DETOXIFYING AND REHYDRATING FRUITS

melon (honeydew, cantaloupe, Ogen, etc.)	peaches	passionfruit
	nectarines	pomegranates
watermelon (91 per cent water)	apricots	cherries
grapes	apples	raspberries
grapefruit	pears	strawberries
pineapple	kiwi fruit	blackberries
oranges	mangoes	blackcurrants
tangerines	pawpaws	redcurrants

For your cooked meals, focus on a carbohydrate – pasta, rice or couscous. Avoid animal fats (meat, cheese, butter and cream), using vegetables, lean chicken (no skin), fish and seafood instead. Any of the meals from the Weekend Programme (see pp. 104–19) are suitable, and here are a few more suggestions.

SPICY FISH SOUP

This makes enough for two servings – if it is just for you, freeze the rest for another day.

6oz/175g white fish

1oz/125g wholemeal flour

1 teaspoon tamari (Japanese soy sauce, available at health-food stores)

1 teaspoon olive oil

juice of $1/2$ a lemon

4oz/100g turnips

1pt/600ml vegetable stock

1 onion, sliced

4oz/100g fennel

pinch of cayenne pepper

Remove the skin from the raw fish and slice it into chunks. In a dish, mix together the flour, tamari, olive oil, lemon juice and, if necessary, a little water so that it forms a smooth paste. If the turnips are thin-skinned, scrub them – otherwise peel them. Chop them into cubes, then put them in a saucepan of boiling vegetable stock and simmer for 5 minutes. Add the sliced onion, fennel and cayenne and simmer for a further 10 minutes. Add the paste, stirring it in until it is well combined. Finally, add the fish and simmer very gently for 10–15 minutes. Serve at once.

VEGETABLE CURRY

This recipe also serves two but, again, it can be frozen or kept in the refrigerator for the next day. Serve with brown or basmati rice.

1 onion

2 tablespoons olive oil

1 teaspoon each of coriander and turmeric

$1/2$ teaspoon curry powder

1 teaspoon root ginger, chopped

1 garlic clove, crushed

2 carrots, sliced

4oz/100g Jerusalem artichokes, sliced

$1/4$pt/150ml vegetable stock

6oz/175g courgettes, sliced

6oz/175g broccoli or cauliflower florets

2oz/50g roasted cashews or almonds

4 tablespoons natural yoghurt

Chop the onion and cook in the olive oil in a large pan until soft. Add the spices, ginger and crushed garlic, then the sliced carrots and Jerusalem artichokes. Cook, stirring, for 2 minutes, then add the stock. Cover and simmer for 10 minutes, then add the sliced courgettes and the broccoli or cauliflower broken into florets. Cook for another 10 minutes. Stir in the nuts. Serve and spoon over the yoghurt.

WEEK TWO

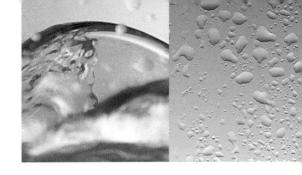

Although the detoxification process of Week One is over, the better your diet for the next 4 weeks, the more benefits that first week will yield. So try to have at least one fruit or vegetable/salad meal each day, and keep your other meals healthy, too – pasta, rice, baked potatoes, grilled fish and lean meat, vegetable stews and soups are all ideal.

For breakfast, Bircher-Benner muesli, stewed dried fruits and porridge all make an excellent start to the day. If you want to go back to drinking tea and coffee, try to limit yourself to one cup a day and substitute herbal teas the rest of the time, but avoid alcohol for at least one more week. Above all, keep your water intake at the same level as last week, with 8 glasses every day.

Exercise

The second week of the programme is a good time to introduce a regular exercise routine into your life if you do not have one already. This does not have to be relentlessly vigorous and, if you are not used to regular exercise, you should certainly start yourself off very gently. Walking, swimming and yoga are all ideal forms of exercise and a combination of the three works best of all.

Walking – providing it is brisk – and swimming are the best forms of aerobic exercise as they have no (or low) impact and so do not put you at risk of injury. What you are aiming at is a 20–30 minute session at least 3 times a week. If you choose walking, you could easily do it more often than this, simply by incorporating it as part

of your journey to work or shopping. Alternatively, head for your local park for a regular, brisk walk and enjoy the scenery as you go.

Swimming is one of the safest forms of exercise as it involves no impact at all. You could also combine a swimming session with a water aerobics class, or with a sauna or a steam. For swimming to be aerobic, however, you must raise your heartbeat sufficiently to make you slightly out of breath – so you cannot take it too easily.

Yoga is non-aerobic, but it is both stretching and strengthening. It may seem as if nothing much is happening, but holding a pose for a minute or two can be surprisingly hard work! Two sets of yoga exercises are given as part of the Weekend Programme (see pp. 108–9 and 115) and, if you combine all of these together, they make a good longer session, ideal for doing several times a week or, even better, daily.

Many people find that just 10–15 minutes of yoga first thing in the morning loosens them up and relaxes them for the entire day. If you do take up yoga, it is really best to find yourself a good teacher to start off with. You will then have a much longer session, learn some new exercises and have your bad habits (and we all have them!) corrected, so that you can get more out of your home sessions.

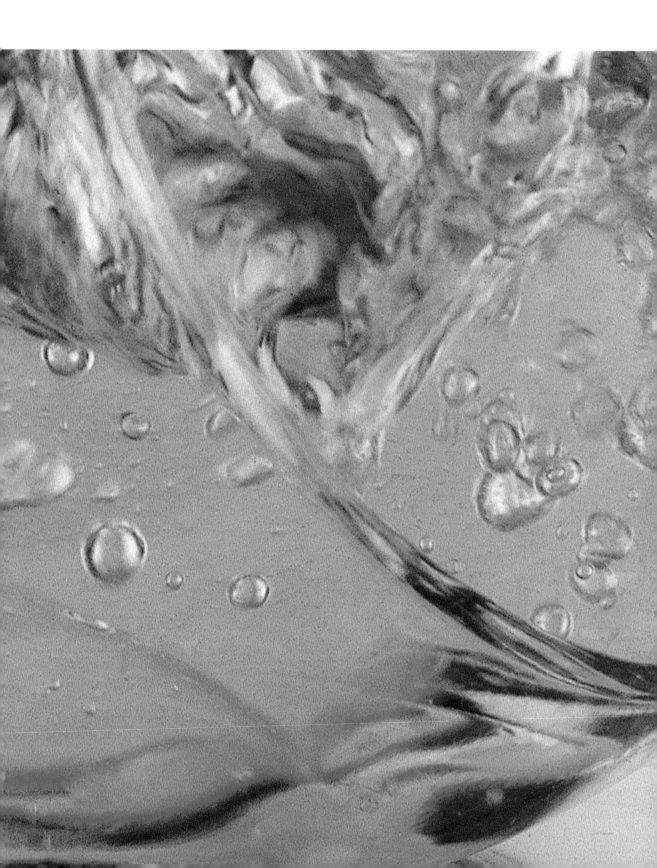

SALUTE TO THE SUN

You could make this the start of your yoga routine, followed by the exercises from the Weekend Programme. This is one of my favourite yoga sequences and perfect for waking you up in the morning, as it stretches out every part of you, simultaneously stimulating the internal organs and the systems of the body.

1   Stand with your feet together and a straight spine, your head held on a long, relaxed neck and your hands together in the prayer position, level with your chest. Take 3 long, deep breaths.

2. On the last out-breath, stretch your arms over your head and, if you can, lean back slightly so that you are looking up at the ceiling (do not lean back if you have a bad back). Then, with your arms still outstretched, breathe in and come back to a standing position. Breathe out and carry on with your arms stretched in front of you, bending from the waist. Try to keep your spine and your arms in the same straight line.

3   Take your hands as close as you can to the floor, letting your head drop right down and your back stretch out. If your hands do not reach the floor, bend your knees until they do.

4   Breathe in and take your right leg straight out behind you, bending your left knee as you do so. Keep your hands on the floor and try to look upwards to the ceiling.

5   Breathe out and take your left leg back, so that the feet are together and your weight is resting on your arms (as if you are in the 'up' stage of a press-up).

6   Breathe in and push your bottom up, so that you are in the dog pose (see p. 115). Breathe out, drop your knees to the floor and lower your chest so that it is also on the floor.

7   Breathe in, then push up on your arms so that your chest comes up and your hips rest on the floor. If you can, turn your face to look upwards.

8   Breathe out and lift your bottom up so that you are in the dog pose again. Then breathe in and bring your right leg forward, bending it at the knee, leaving your left leg stretched out behind you. If you can, look up and breathe out.

9   Breathe in and bring your left foot to meet the right, with your hands still on the floor – bend your knees, if necessary. Breathe out. Then breathe in again and, with your arms outstretched and a straight back, come back to the standing position, bending from the hips.

10 Breathe out and return to the prayer position. You can repeat this sequence several times, and you will speed up as you become familiar with it. However, always make sure that you really *feel* the stretch of every position.

RELAXATION

At the end of a yoga session always do a short relaxation. Lie down on the floor and cover yourself, as your temperature drops during relaxation. Let your arms lie a little apart from your body, palms facing upwards, and let your legs roll away from each other until there is no tension in them (in yoga, this is known as the corpse position!). Close your eyes and make sure that your neck is long and that there is no tension in your neck or shoulders. Take a few long, deep breaths and feel your body lying heavily on the floor.

Now, working upwards from the toes, focus on each part of the body in turn, feeling it soften and relax. From the toes, move upwards through the calves and knees to the thighs. Then feel the heaviness of your legs on the floor. Then let your focus move through the buttocks, the hips and the abdomen. As you release the abdomen you may feel the lower spine soften, too, and get closer to the floor.

Continue moving your focus upwards through the stomach, the waist and the chest, then into the shoulders and down through the arms, right to the fingertips. Now bring the focus back to the neck, the back of the head and the face (which often carries a great deal of tension). Lie like this for 5 minutes, just enjoying the feeling of relaxation. Then take a deep breath in and appreciate the sensation of your body becoming awake again and aware of its surroundings. Wriggle your fingers and toes, stretch your arms and legs and, when you are ready, roll on to your side, open your eyes and get up very slowly.

MEDITATION

Meditation is a wonderful antidote to stress and tiredness and, by stilling the mind on a regular basis, you seem to enhance its functions. There is a growing body of evidence to show that meditation enhances concentration, alertness and creativity. Its physical effects are equally wide-ranging, and it has been shown that meditation lowers blood pressure and improves the circulation; research is currently under way into whether meditation can also affect cancer.

MEDITATION TECHNIQUES

Meditation may take a number of forms. One is visualization (see also pp. 8–9), which you can do by yourself or using a tape to help you get started. Other easy techniques to learn are breathing meditation and using a mantra.

Visualization involves picturing a scene in your mind. Start by sitting calmly and quietly, focusing on your breathing. Either imagine a place or picture somewhere with which you are familiar, then add some water to it, perhaps in the form of a lake or fountain; alternatively use an audio tape to help you visualize and hear waves crashing on to a beach, or the sound of sea creatures. Focus on the movement of the water, as it ripples, cascades or crashes; count the waves as they break; or concentrate on the sound made by the water or by the creatures.

Breathing meditation focuses on the breath itself. Place your attention on your breathing and, as you breathe in, count one. As you breathe out, count two, and so on. Every time you forget to count – or find yourself thinking about something else – go back to one and start again.

A mantra is simply a symbolic word that you repeat. The best-known mantra is 'Om' (pronounced 'Aum'), and you repeat it mentally as you breathe out. You are aiming to let your whole mind fill with its sound and resonance. If 'Om' does not appeal to you, then choose a word that has special significance for you.

Do not expect to be able to meditate without other thoughts coming into your mind – it takes years to get to that stage and few people actually manage it! Just put the thoughts to one side to deal with later, if necessary, and gently bring your focus back to your image, your breathing or the mantra. After the session sit quietly for a few minutes, trying to instil yourself for the remainder of the day with the tranquillity you have created. Start with a 10-minute session and, if you wish, build up to 20. Do one or two sessions every day, preferably at the same time.

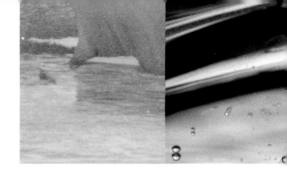

WEEK FOUR

By this stage in the programme you should be feeling significantly better than you did at its start. Your body will certainly be rehydrated and will have rid itself of many residual toxins. If you continue with the same high water intake and healthy diet, with plenty of fresh fruit and vegetables, these benefits will increase over the weeks and months to come, particularly if you also include some of the other elements of the programme – exercise, hydrotherapy, meditation – as part of your daily routine. Obviously, no one will keep religiously to any routine, and everyone has occasional lapses. Just think of Christmas! The important thing is to return to a healthy diet as soon as you can. In the meantime, keep drinking copious quantities of water.

The first three weeks of the programme have dealt mostly with what you can do internally – whether this concerns your digestive system, your liver, your muscles or your mind – to improve your health and well-being. This final week looks at external improvements, and in particular at your environment.

ARID ENVIRONMENTS

We nearly all live and work in highly unnatural environments. Our homes and offices are often insulated and overheated and this, in turn, means that they have very low humidity. Air conditioning dries out the air and electronic equipment, such as computers and photocopiers, produces its own additional dry heat. The air we are breathing becomes increasingly dry and relative humidity commonly stands at around 25 per cent, which is the same as that of the Sahara Desert. And hot, dry air is greedy for moisture. It will take it from anywhere it can get it: plants, furniture and, of course, you.

If dry air can, over time, split the wood of furniture, imagine what it can do to your body. The most common problems are headaches and dry eyes (and this can be a severe problem if you wear contact lenses), shocks from static electricity, skin problems such as eczema, and the exacerbation of respiratory complaints such as colds, laryngitis, sore throats and bronchitis. The respiratory system functions smoothly only by means of its watery mucus and, if this is dried out due to low relative humidity, it becomes thicker and more sluggish. Dirt and germs get stuck in the system, instead of being flushed straight through, and infections can therefore take hold more easily. You may often feel as if you are getting a cold, even if you are not; if you do have a cold, your symptoms feel even worse.

Low humidity has a bad effect on the skin, too. As the dry air leaches water from the top layer of your skin, it is forced to draw more and more water from the dermis and the hypodermis beneath – and this is, of

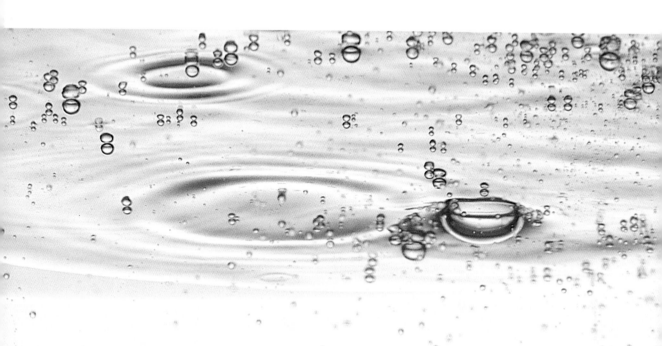

course, even more of a problem if you are dehydrated yourself. Over time, the skin visibly dries out and, as we already know, dry skin ages more quickly (see pp. 48–9), developing fine lines and wrinkles.

MOISTENING THE ATMOSPHERE

The 'comfort zone' for relative humidity is 50–55 per cent. This means that you need to find a way of bringing more moisture into your living or working space. Fish tanks, vases of flowers and plants all help in yielding some moisture to the air, but the only efficient way of keeping the atmosphere balanced is by using a humidifier.

HUMIDIFIERS

There are two basic types:

Non-electric humidifiers are very inexpensive and, of course, silent. There are various models that you can hang on a radiator or place on top of a storage heater, double-width radiator or gas fire. The working principle is simple – the hot surface of the radiator makes the humidifier's water evaporate into the air. Such humidifiers need to be filled with fresh water every day. You can add aromatherapy oils to the water, too, for a therapeutic or scented effect.

Electric humidifiers are more powerful and often include other functions, like purifying (to counteract airborne pollution, such as cigarette smoke, pollen, soot and exhaust fumes) or ionizing the air. (Ionized air contains a higher proportion of negatively charged molecules and has been linked with relief from respiratory disorders and asthma.) Some models produce cool air; some steam; others an ice-cold mist. Some have a built-in hygrostat – like a thermometer for humidity – and will set themselves automatically. Several can be used in conjunction with aromatherapy oils (see Resources on p. 141 for further information).

FACIAL AFFUSIONS

Keeping the relative humidity of your environment at the right level will help to keep the water level in your own skin stable and prevent ageing. Another rejuvenating treatment you could try this week is a facial affusion, which tightens facial skin. This is a bit like a cold shower for the face! However, it is done as a continuing gentle flow of water and the effect is rather like a water massage.

You can use your shower, as long as it is of the flexible hose (rather than rigid pipe) sort – but not a power shower, for the pressure would be too great. You need to take off the shower head, so that you are using just the mouth of the hose. A good time to do this is at the end of your bath, when you can rest your head against the back of the bath. Hold the shower hose a few inches from your face so that the water will flow over it in a smooth stream. Then move the hose as slowly as you can so that the water circles your face: 3 times clockwise, then 3 times anticlockwise. Then take the water slowly from side to side of your forehead, three times, resting for a moment at each temple and again in the centre. Take the hose slowly around the jawline, from side to side, again 3 times. Finish with 3 water circles in each direction.

FACING THE FUTURE

The end of Week Four represents the end of the One-Month Programme. However, I hope there will be some elements that you have found sufficiently beneficial that you will want to continue them in your normal day-to-

day routine. The single most important one is, of course, keeping your daily water intake up to 8 glasses a day. A healthy diet and regular exercise are, as we all know, vital to our well-being, and many of the treatments and therapies that you can do yourself at home have long-lasting benefits for everything from your immune function to the way you look.

Water has been cleansing, refreshing and purifying people for millennia. Whether you are drinking it, bathing in it, swimming in it, steaming in it, showering in it or meditating on it, it is one of our last great free resources. Enjoy it.

ASIA

CHIVA SOM
73-4 Petchkasem Road
Hua Hin 77110
Thailand
Tel: (66) 325 365 36

A luxurious spa in a breathtaking setting – built to look like a traditional Thai village – with a combination of Western hydrotherapy, rejuvenation programmes and ancient Eastern therapies and philosophy.

JAVANA SPA
Jakarta
Java
Indonesia
Tel: (662) 171 983 27

This Javanese spa is located in a lush rainforest on the slopes of a volcanic mountain. The day begins wtih a walk through the mountain clouds to a waterfall bath, and continues through a day of body treatments to On-Sen, an evening traditional sulphu bath.

AUSTRALIA

CONRAN COVE RESORT
Conran Cove
Australia
Tel: (61) 755 979 00

An eco-spa surrounded by water – in fact, you get there by water taxi. The facilities here are mostly water-based on Spa Island. There is a wide range of treatments and far more water in its natural state. You can also walk through the rainforest with a native guide.

USA

THE BROADMOOR
1 Lake Avenue
Colorado Springs
Colorado 80906
Tel: (1) 800 634 7711

A world-class spa in the Rockies, the Broadmoor uses mountain water for cascading showers, relaxing baths and whirlpools, Vichy showers, indoor and outdoor pools and a range of hydrotherapy treatments.

THE SPA INTERNAZIONALE AT FISHER ISLAND
1 Fisher Island Drive
Fisher Island
Miami 33109
Florida
Tel: (1) 800 537 3708

A car-free island spa that houses only 10 guests at a time, Fisher Island has indoor and outdoor pools, hydroptherapy and body treatments as well as yoga, golf and tennis.

TWO BUNCH PALMS
67-425 Two Bunch Palms
   Trail
Desert Hot Springs
California
Tel: (1) 760 329 8791

Another luxurious spa, with each of its private cabins coming with its own jacuzzi. Built on a geological fault, it has its own hot spring, and offers underwater massage and many other hydrotherapy treatments.

Spas can be booked through the Spa Directory, New York, USA
Tel: (1) 212 924 6800
Fax: (1) 212 924 7240
www.spafinders.com

RESOURCES

AYUVERDIC HEALTH CARE AND SILK GLOVES FOR SKIN-BRUSHING

European Ayurveda
Hoar Cross Hall
Hoar Cross
Nr Yoxall
Staffordshire DE13 8QS
Tel: 01283 576 515
www.europeanayurveda.com

IMPLOSION RESEARCH

Centre for Implosion Research
PO Box 38
Plymouth
Devon PL7 5YX
Tel: 01752 345 552
Fax: 01752 338 569

FLOTATION TANKS

Float Works
Winchester Wharf
Clink Street
London SE1 9DG
Tel: 0207 357 0111

WATER FILTERS

Fresh Water Filter Manufacturing
Carlton House
Aylmer Road
Leytonstone
London E11 3AD
Tel: 0208 558 7495
Fax: 0208 556 9270

HUMIDIFIERS

Air Improvement Centre
23 Denbigh Street
London SW1V 2HF
Tel: 0207 834 2834
Fax: 0207 630 8485

HYDROTHERM MASSAGE

For details of local therapists call 01296 714 254